Box Set

Natural Body Scrubs At Home

&

Natural Body Detox

By

Laura Serio

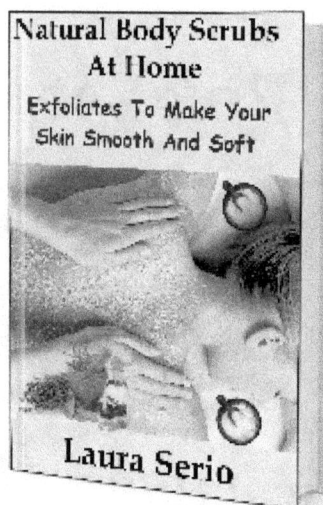

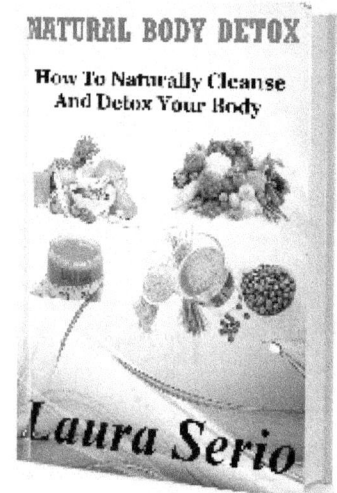

First of all I would like to thank you and congratulate for purchasing this Box Set. I hope you will enjoy reading these books!!

Book 1

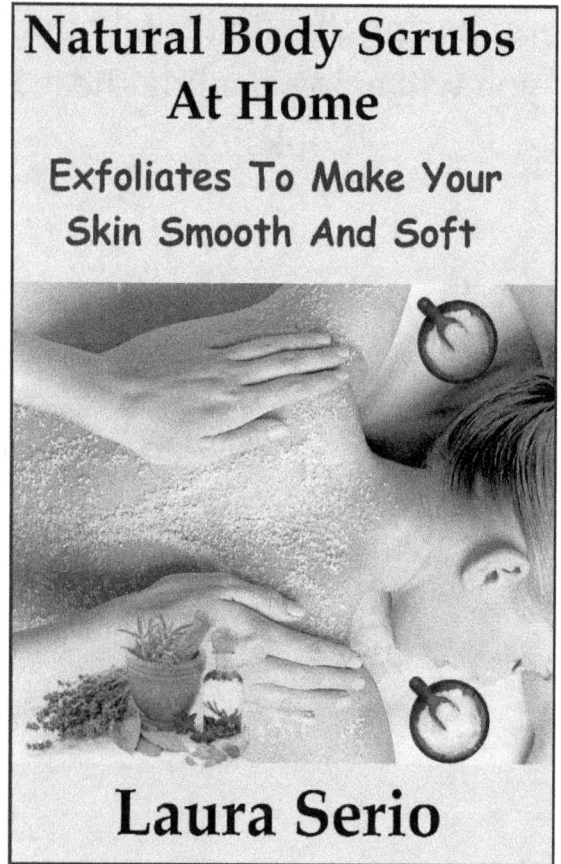

Natural Body Scrubs
At Home

Exfoliates To Make Your
Skin Smooth And Soft

Laura Serio

Natural Body Scrubs At Home

Exfoliates To Make Your Skin Smooth And Soft

By

Laura Serio

Laura Serio

informational purposes only and presented "as is" without warranty or guarantee of any kind.

ACKNOWLEDGMENTS

For my students and friends, who all selflessly helped me in writing this book. Special thanks to those who asked, insisted and assisted me in turning the seminars in this practical form. All Rights Reserved 2012-2015 @ Laura Serio.

Laura Serio

Table of Contents

Natural Body Scrubs At Home

INTRODUCTION

We all are so much concerned about of skin and beauty. Using ready-made beauty product is the one thing, which people prefer these days to improve their looks, but these products include so many chemicals, which are sometimes harmful for our health and skin. And so it is always good to use natural body scrubs or homemade products for your skin.

Here in this book, I am going to share with you all natural scrubs recipes that you can make in your home. These recipes are perfect to improve your beauty and to make your skin glowing. Using body scrubs will provide your body a means of exfoliation. It is a process that rids of old skin from the body and enables the new skin to rise.

Overall body scrubs helped you rejuvenate your skin regularly. I tried all these scrubs recipes at my home, with my friends and relatives. After seeing the results and benefits, I thought to write a book about natural scrubs, so that I can share it will you all. I am sure you will be benefitted from it.

I hope this book will help you to create your own beauty products. Try them at share your reviews with me. Thanks for purchasing the book.

WHAT ARE BODY SCRUBS?

A body scrub is in general a body treatment which is similar to a facial, like we do face facial, similarly with body scrub we can do body facial. It is basically done because it exfoliates and hydrates your skin, leaving it smooth and soft. Mostly for body scrub an abrasive material like salt, sugar, coffee grounds, rice bran, even pecan hulls, is used which is mixed with some kind of massage oil and an aromatic essential oils.

Body scrubs are best to keep your skin healthy and beautiful through exfoliation. Exfoliant is an abrasive material which rubs away the dead skin cells on the surface, revealing the softer, younger cells. Today there are so many therapists and massage centers, which provide body scrubs. You can go to their centers for body scrubs, or you can purchase body scrubs and can scrub your body at home, or you can make your own scrub at home and can scrub your body.

Body scrubs mainly contain skin-nourishing ingredients and chemical Exfoliants to dissolve the intracellular "glue" that holds cells together. Body scrubs which are available at spa centers are more thorough and leave your skin softer. Working longer with body scrubs gets the chemicals into areas where you can't reach easily.

Things To Consider When Doing Body Scrub From The Therapist:

- A body scrub is usually done in a wet room, which has a tile floor and a drain.

- When body scrub starts, you need to face-down on a massage table that is covered with a towel, a sheet or a thin piece of plastic and a shower overhead.

- The therapist starts body scrub by gently rubbing exfoliates on your back, the backs of your arms, and the backs of your legs and feet.

- When the therapist is finished with this process, you then step into a shower to rinse off.

- While you were showering, therapist put clean sheets on the treatment table.

- Then you dry off and lay face-down on the treatment table under a sheet or towel.

This was all about when you take a body scrub from the therapist, but the great thing is that you can make body scrub at home also. As many of us don't get time to visit a therapist, and some of us feel shy to go for a body scrub. So, here in this book I am sharing with your body scrub recipes that you can easily make in your home. And these are made from all natural ingredients, so they will not harm your skin.

How Often One Should Use Body Scrub?

Using a body scrub is good, but using it on a daily basis is not a good habit. Because frequent scrubbing can damage your skin layer once the dead skin is off the body surface. It's always good to use a body scrub once in a week or thrice a month. Using scrub gently also make your skin dry. Also during winters, too much scrubbing can damage the already dry skin of yours.

HOW TO USE BODY SCRUBS

Here are some tips on how to use body scrubs. These tips will be helpful whether you are using a body scrub for the first time or you are using it often times. Have a look at them-

First of all keep your hair pulled up through the whole process. Otherwise, you might wake up with scrub grinds still in your hair.

Use a mirror Near your tub so that you can easily scrub the grinds on your face without getting any in your eyes or mouth.

Your hands and feet are the important part of the body that needs to spend extra time exfoliating because they get the hardest beating. For feet you need to take extra care, add a pedicure block to help scrub your calluses.

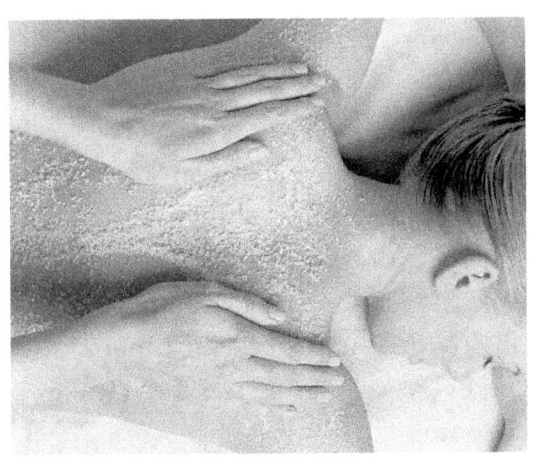

If your skin is healthy and firm, then you can use scrub up to 3 times a week, but if you have sensitive or thin skin, then you must use it once a week.

Hold off on running the water in the shower and then rub your scrub in circular motions with your hand onto dry skin for full and longer-lasting coverage. Now turn on the water and rinse, using your hands to help remove any remaining granules.

If you have a bath tub in your bathroom, then prefer to do scrubbing there only. Don't venture past the tub, else it will be messy. Stay in the shower and it will easily wash down the drain, otherwise, you will be scrambling to sweep the bathroom floors later on.

When you rub, scrub on the body; make sure you do not over scrub, as it will lead your body to irritation. And if you have fair skin, your skin will be red from scrubbing. So, always moisturize your body after you have dried off.

Natural Body Scrubs At Home

After taking bath, prefer to clean your body with a dark color towel, keep your clothes and white towels out of sight.

When using a body scrub make sure to use a wet wash cloth and scrub your entire body from shoulders to feet.

HEALTH BENEFITS OF A BODY SCRUB

A body scrub is basically a suspension of coarse granules such as apricots, walnut, and oatmeal, sea salt in a semi-liquid medium or gel. For maintaining healthy, smooth skin, it is a good idea to use body scrubs. Although many body scrubs are available at retail stores and online stores, but it is always good to use homemade natural body scrubs.

The main purpose of a body scrub is to remove dead skin cells through exfoliation as well as cleanse the skin and increase the body's blood circulation. Here in this book you will learn how body scrub can improve your skin's health. You will also find tips on choosing the best product for your body and how to properly use a scrub to give your skin the invigorating rubdown it craves.

Natural Body Scrubs At Home

Body scrubs help to remove the dead skin layer and expose younger looking supple skin. Our body skin sheds on a regular basis so as to reveal new, healthier skin. This process slows down as we get older, and hence comes the need of a body scrub. A scrub works in many ways like you can massage it over your body. The exfoliating granules in scrub help to slough off dead skin, and the rubbing action boosts the blood circulation and helps drain your lymph nodes.

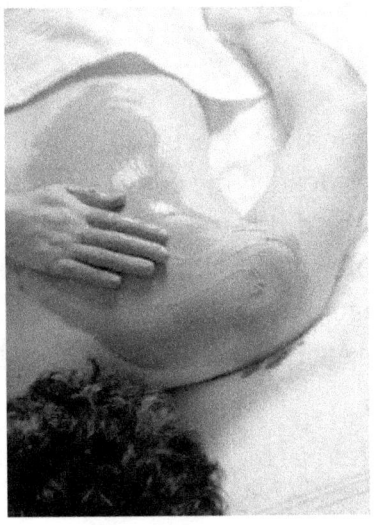

BENEFITS

Makes Skin Look Fresh and Rejuvenated. A body scrub removes dead skin cells from the body and impurities, leaving you feeling fresh and your skin looking rejuvenated and revitalized.

After using scrub you will feel mindful of the refreshing texture against your skin and captivating scent that fills the shower and allows you to enjoy the treatment.

Makes Skin Look More Youthful. It exfoliates dead skin cells and tends to remove the dull and lackluster appearance of the skin. Using a body scrub regularly will help make your skin look more vibrant and youthful.

Natural Body Scrubs At Home

Body scrubs are also great for removing self-tanner from your body. If your skin had become rough and has darkened due to pollution or exposure to dust, you can use a body scrub to remove the rough skin layer leaving you with a soft and supple skin.

It provides great Moisturizing Benefits. Body scrubs benefits through the removal of dead skin cells as a result of exfoliation with a mild body scrub extend to moisturizing as it allows for easier absorption of a skin moisturizer into the healthy skin.

It makes your skin glow, especially with a salt scrub. The results for your body will depend on the type of salt you use.

Using a body scrub encourages the natural flow of blood circulation and bodily fluids within. It is also said that body scrubs can actually improve the look of aging and dimpled skin from cellulite.

If you treat yourself to a body scrub, it is just plain relaxing. Having a body scrub done by a professional gives you more benefit without the mess or stress.

Getting a body scrub done at a spa regularly can be expensive, but there are many options to make your own scrubs at home. With the benefits that body scrubs allow, the effort is worth it.

It is also believed that by body scrubs stimulate the skin and blood circulation and prevents skin disorders, skin disease, and even prevent certain physical ailments.

Natural Body Scrubs At Home

Cleansing your body with scrub opens pores and cleanses them. By opening the pores you allow your skin to breathe and to excrete oils that can build up and cause not only oily skin, but acne or blackheads as well.

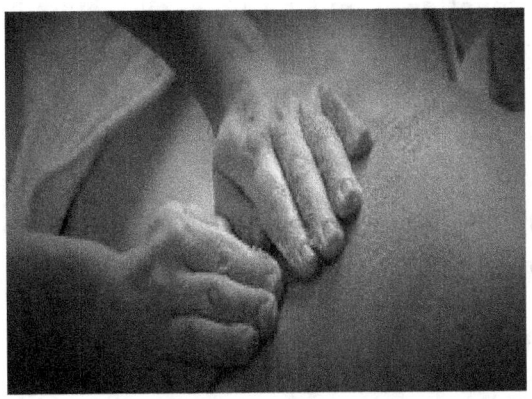

It makes your skin looks and feels young. It also prevents you to stay away from cellulite and age spots. By using a body scrub you can help your skin to be more youthful and more attractive.

DIFFERENCE BETWEEN MANUAL AND CHEMICAL EXFOLIATING SCRUBS

Exfoliating basically helps to remove dead skin cells from the surface of your skin, and keeps your skin fresh and healthy. Exfoliation stimulates new cell growth by removing the cells your body is no longer shedding. It helps your body with the desquamation process by stripping the dead epidermal cells on the outer surface of your skin and exposing a fresher layer of living cells.

It takes a few days for a noticeable amount of dead cells to accumulate. It is best to exfoliate once or twice a week. You don't want to irritate your skin or remove healthy living cells by doing it daily. In general there are two types of exfoliation: manual or physical and chemical exfoliates.

Manual or Physical

Manual exfoliation is when you scrub your skin yourself. This scrub could be a homemade scrub, or even a simple washcloth. You can make your own scrub at home by adding coffee, sugar or baking soda to few other products and physically scrub your body.

Physically exfoliates removes dead cells through friction. Manual exfoliation is moved across your skin's surface using your fingers or buff puff. Dead cells are removed by scraping off the top surface with physical friction. Most of the manufacturers use natural products such as seeds, apricot pits, or crushed oyster shells as the ingredient in the scrubs, because these ingredients are good for causing friction.

Chemical

Chemical exfoliation is the one in which exfoliating is done with chemicals that help shield your skin faster. This can be in the form of a serum, toner, treatment, product, or chemical peel. Mainly in chemical exfoliation acids are used.

Chemical exfoliates to remove dead skin cells by dissolving the "glue" that binds them to other cells. They are a topical ingredient that can dissolve the glue like substance that holds the dead cells together. Most chemicals exfoliate either use Alpha Hydroxy Acids or Beta Hydroxy Acids. This type of exfoliation is applied to the skin, and then rinsed off. You do no "scrub" to enjoy the benefits; the chemical does the entire job.

HOMEMADE EXFOLIATES INGREDIENTS

All the body scrubs (exfoliates) which are made at home mostly consists of three ingredients, namely an exfoliate, carrier oil and a fragrance. We will have a look at them in deep:

1. An Exfoliate

It is a gritty substance used in scrubs. Most commonly used exfoliate are Sugar and salt as they can be easily dissolved in water and don't leave any mess in your bathtub. Salt is best for relaxing your muscles and it has been said that using sea salt is better than using table salt, as it contains a wider variety of trace elements and minerals, and is good for the skin. While sugar is lightly gentler on your skin as compared to salt. You can use either brown or white sugar.

Apart from sugar and salt, another exfoliate used is coffee. Coffee smells divine, and the caffeine has its own benefits for your skin. Caffeine is a vasoconstrictor, which means it causes blood vessels to constrict, so it reduces varicose veins and resources. Oatmeal is another gentle exfoliates, which is an emollient, meaning that it softens and hydrates your skin. It has been used for decades as an effective home remedy for dry and itchy skin. Few others commonly use exfoliates are almond meal, flax meal, rice bran, wheat bran, and groundnut shells.

2. Carrier Oil

Carrier oil is also known as base oil. This oil is used in homemade body scrub to hold the mixture together, and to moisturize your skin. There are many carrier oils available in the market. Some of the popular carrier oils are Sunflower oil, which has a very faint odor, thin consistency, and penetrates well without leaving much of a residue. It is one of the most affordable oils and has a shelf life of about 12 months. Sweet Almond Oil has a slightly sweet and nutty aroma, medium consistency, and absorbs fairly quickly with Shelf life of about 12 months.

Grape Seed Oil has a faint sweet odor, is very thin, and leaves a thin film on the skin with a shelf life of 6-12 months. Hazelnut Oil has a sweet, nutty odor, is quite thin, and leaves a film on the skin with a Shelf life of about 12 months.

Apart from these few other carrier oils which are commonly used are Kukui Oil, Macadamia Nut Oil, and a lot more.

3. Fragrance

The best way to scent your homemade scrub is to use essential oils. Remember fragrance oils are synthetic, so avoid them and use essential oils instead. Here are some commonly used essential oil, namely lavender oil, sandalwood oil, chamomile oil, rose oil, Neroli oil, geranium oil, etc. remember to avoid getting undiluted essential oil on your skin - it is very concentrated and can cause irritation. For sensitive skin, avoid the following oils: basil, cinnamon, clove, lemon, lemongrass, tea-tree, and thyme, citrus.

Now, as you know the basic ingredients, you can make your own recipes for homemade body scrubs. Let's have a look at few starter recipes for you.

HOMEMADE NATURAL BODY SCRUBS

Sugar Scrub Recipes

Sugar scrub is the best, effective and inexpensive scrub to make easily at home. It is a simple beauty recipe with countless variations, and is can be incredibly moisturizing and exfoliating of the skin. It can be used on face, body, and feet. It is best for silky skin. It takes around 5-10 minutes to prepare sugar scrub recipe, and it's great for exfoliating skin naturally.

Pumpkin Sugar Scrub

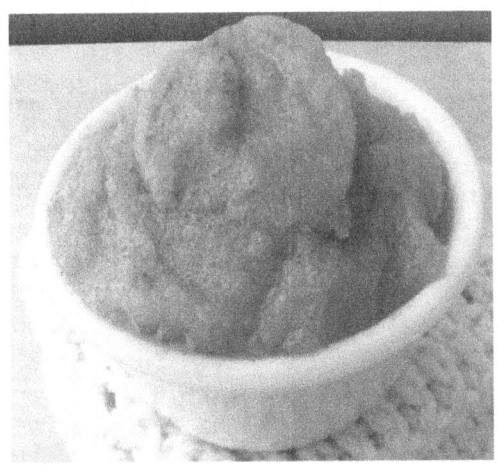

Ingredients required

½ cup of sugar

¼ cup of coconut oil

½ tsp essential oil

½ tsp pumpkin

Instructions

Take a bowl and add sugar, pumpkin and coconut oil. Stir it thoroughly.

Add essential oil continue stirring. Stop when the scrub reaches the consistency of moist sand. Store it in an air tight jar.

Whenever you need to scrub your body, take 1 tablespoon as needed in the shower. Scrub your skin with the mixture and rinse well.

It will leave your skin smooth and silky.

<u>Vanilla Sugar Scrub</u>

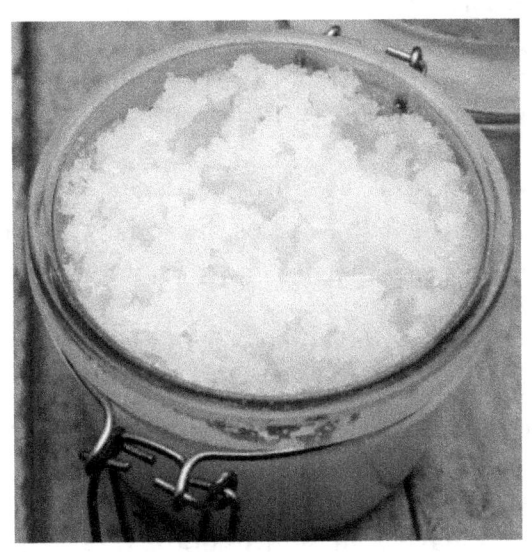

Ingredients required

½ cup of sugar

¼ cup of almond oil

½ tsp essential oil

½ tsp vanilla extract

Instructions

Take a bowl and add sugar, vanilla extract and almond oil. Stir it thoroughly.

Add essential oil continue stirring. Stop when the scrub reaches the consistency of moist sand. Store it in an air tight jar.

Whenever you need to scrub your body, take 1 tablespoon as needed in the shower. Scrub your skin with the mixture and rinse well.

It will leave your skin smooth and silky.

<u>Lemon Sugar Scrub</u>

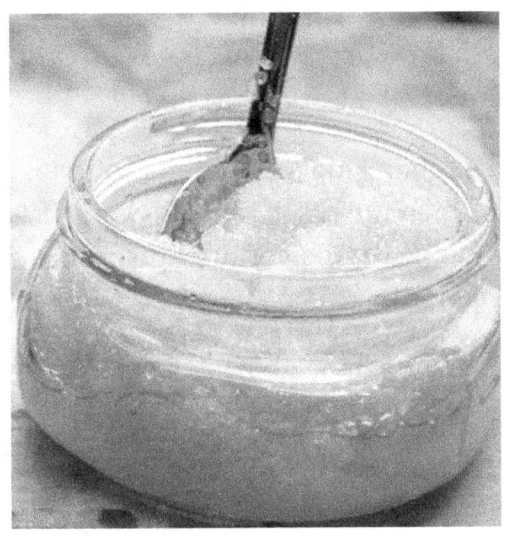

Ingredients required

½ cup of sugar

¼ cup of almond oil

½ tsp Vitamin E oil

1-2 tsp of lemon drops

Instructions

Take a bowl and add sugar, lemon drops and almond oil. Stir it thoroughly.

Add vitamin E oil and continue stirring. Stop when the scrub reaches the consistence of moist sand. Store it in an air tight jar.

Whenever you need to scrub your body, take 1 tablespoon as needed in the shower. Scrub your skin with the mixture and rinse well.

It will leave your skin smooth and silky.

<u>Vanilla Lavender Sugar Scrub</u>

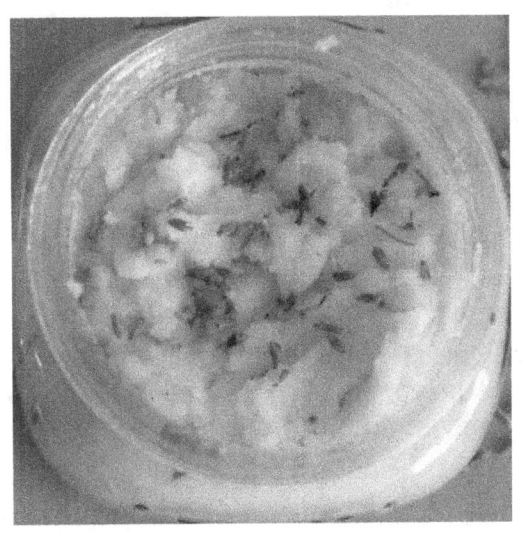

Ingredients required

½ cup of sugar

¼ cup of almond oil

½ tsp Vitamin E oil

½ tsp vanilla extract

½ tsp Lavender essential oil

Instructions

Take a bowl and add sugar, almond oil, lavender oil and vanilla extract. Stir it thoroughly.

Add Vitamin E oil and continue stirring. Stop when the scrub reaches the consistency of moist sand. Store it in an air tight jar.

Whenever you need to scrub your body, take 1 tablespoon as needed in the shower. Scrub your skin with the mixture and rinse well.

It will leave your skin smooth and silky.

<u>Peppermint Sugar Scrub</u>

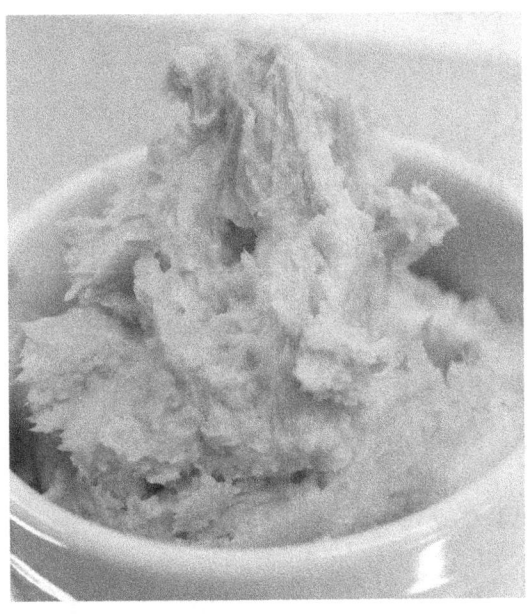

Ingredient Required

1/4 cup coconut oil

1/2 cup melts and pours soap

3-4 drops of peppermint essential oil

1 cup sugar

Instructions

Take a boiler and melt your shredded soap in it and stir in between until melted.

Now in a bowl add coconut oil and peppermint essential oil to the melted soap.

Add sugar to the bowl, and mix until well combined.

Let it dry for 1-2 hours and your peppermint scrub is ready.

Whenever you need to scrub your body, take 1 tablespoon as needed in the shower. Scrub your skin with the mixture and rinse well.

It will leave your skin smooth and silky.

<u>Gingerbread Sugar Scrub</u>

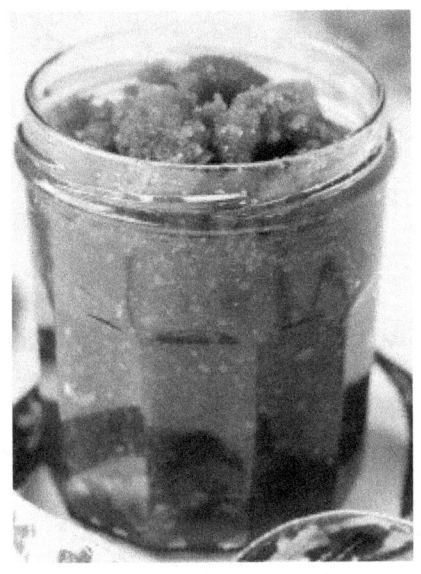

Ingredient Required

1 cup sugar

1 cup brown sugar

1/2 cup coconut oil

1/4 cup almond oil

1/2 tsp vanilla extract

1/2 tsp cinnamon

1/2 tsp all spice

1/2 tsp ginger

1/2 tsp nutmeg

Instructions

In a bowl mix all the ingredients except oils.

Now gradually add coconut & almond oil until the scrub reaches desired consistency.

Pour it into an air tight container and your scrub is ready.

Whenever you need to scrub your body, take 1 tablespoon as needed in the shower. Scrub your skin with the mixture and rinse well.

It will leave your skin smooth and silky.

Lemon & Honey Sugar Scrub

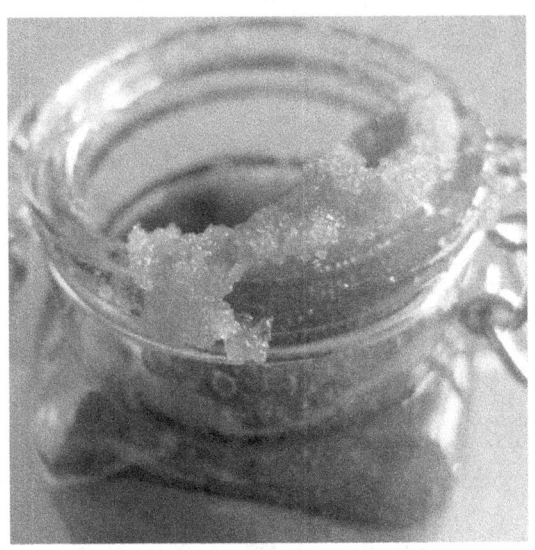

Ingredient Required

1 cup organic cane sugar

1/4 cup olive oil

2 tsp honey

2 tsp dried rosemary

15 drops lemon essential oil

15 drops lavender essential oil

Instructions

Take a bowl and mix sugar, dried rosemary, olive oil, and raw honey well.

Now add essential oils and stir to combine.

Your scrub is ready; store it into an air tight container.

Whenever you need to scrub your body, take 1 tablespoon as needed in the shower. Scrub your skin with the mixture and rinse well.

It will leave your skin smooth and silky.

<u>Peach Tea Sugar Scrub</u>

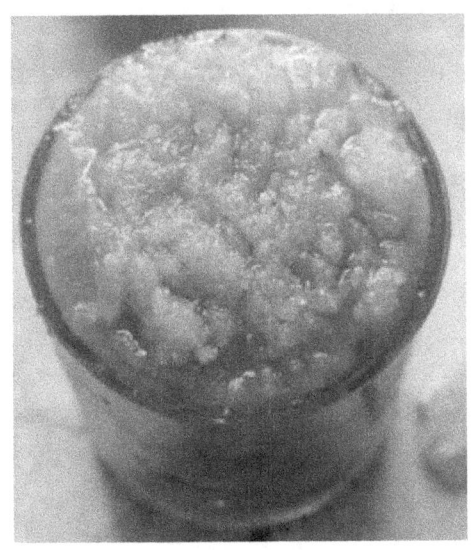

Ingredients Required

1 ½ cups sugar

½- ¾ cup coconut oil

4-5 peach tea bags

Essential oils

Instructions

Open peach tea bags empty leaves and keep it aside.

In a bowl take sugar, loose tea leaves and mixes all there ingredients well.

Slowly add coconut oil and stir until all the mixture is covered in oil.

Place in air tight container and your scrub is ready.

Whenever you need to scrub your body, take 1 tablespoon as needed in the shower. Scrub your skin with the mixture and rinse well.

It will leave your skin smooth and silky.

<u>Green Tea Sugar Scrub</u>

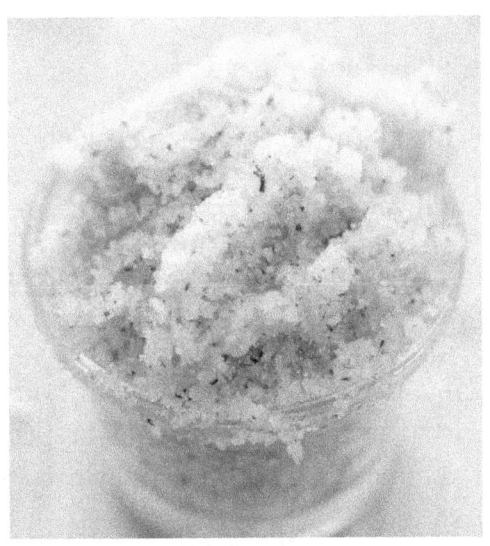

Ingredients Required

1 Cup Granulated Sugar

1/8 Cup Grape seed Oil

1/8 Cup Brewed Green Tea

1 Bag Green Tea

Instructions

Take a bowl and add sugar to it.

Now mix all the oil to the sugar well.

Gradually add green tea and stirrer well.

Make a thick paste and store it in air tight container. Your scrub is ready.

Whenever you need to scrub your body, take 1 tsp as needed in the shower. Scrub your skin with the mixture and rinse well.

It will leave your skin smooth and silky.

Chocolate Coconut Sugar Scrub

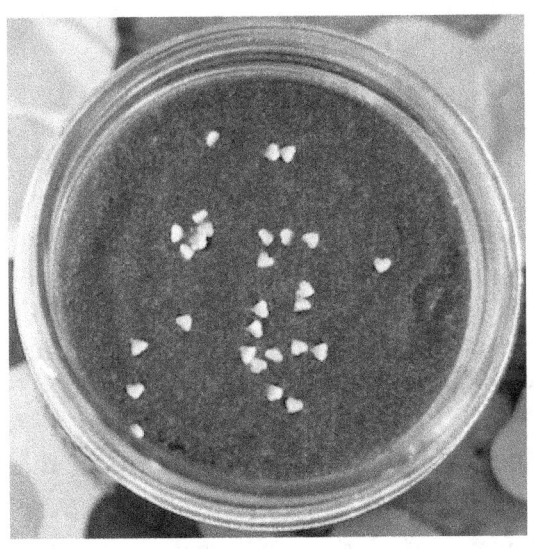

Ingredients Required

1 cup sugar

1/2 cup coconut oil

1/3 cup almond oil

2 tsps cocoa powder

20 drops of coconut extract or essential oil

Instructions

Take a bowl and mix all the ingredients well.

Mix it with the back of a spoon until no chunks remain.

Scrub is ready; store it in a tight container at room temperature.

Whenever you need to scrub your body, take 1 tsp as needed in the shower. Scrub your skin with the mixture and rinse well.

It will leave your skin smooth and silky.

Banana Sugar Scrub

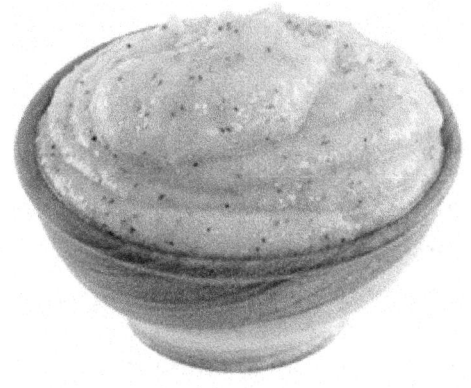

Ingredients Required

1 ripe banana

3 tsps granulated sugar

¼ tsp vanilla extract

1 tsp essential oil

Instructions

Take a bowl and with a fork smash the banana. Doesn't over-mash or it will become too thin?

Mix all the ingredients in the bowl and add essential oil gradually.

Your banana scrub is ready. Gently massage over your body.

Whenever you need to scrub your body, take 1 tsp as needed in the shower. Scrub your skin with the mixture and rinse well.

It will leave your skin smooth and silky.

Vanilla Coconut Brown Sugar Scrub

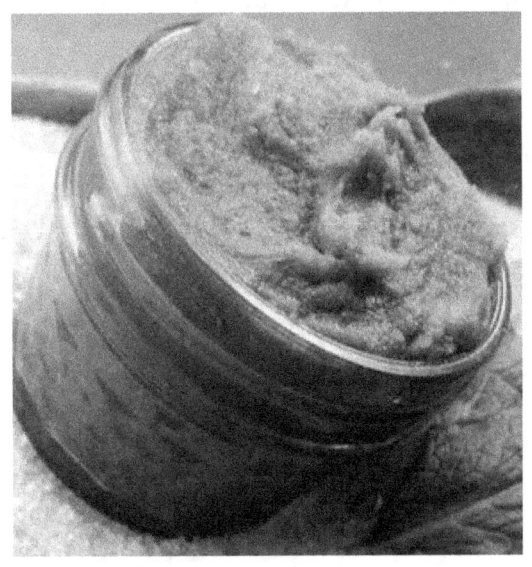

Ingredients Required

1/2 cup coconut oil

1/2 cup brown sugar

1/2 teaspoon vanilla

Instructions

Take a bowl and mix all the ingredients in it.

Your scrub is ready; store it in air tight container at room temperature.

Whenever you need to scrub your body, take 1 tsp as needed in the shower. Scrub your skin with the mixture and rinse well.

It will leave your skin smooth and silky.

Salt Scrub Recipes

<u>Grapefruit Salt Scrub</u>

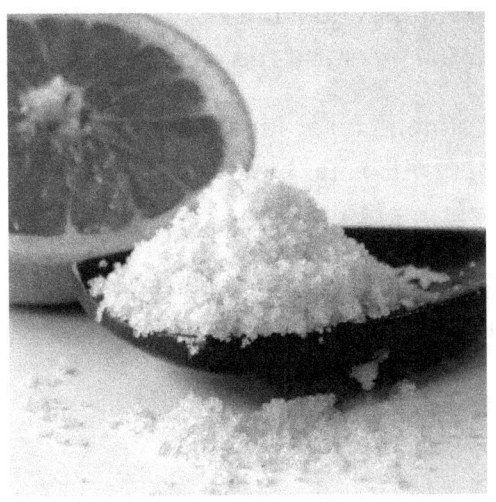

Ingredients required

1 cup salt

1/3 cup almond oil

8 drops grapefruit essential oil

8 bergamot

4 peppermints

Instructions

Take a bowl and add salt to grapefruit essential oil. Stir it thoroughly.

Add almond oil gradually and continue stirring. Also add bergamot and peppermint to it.

Stop when the scrub reaches the consistency of moist sand.

Your scrub is ready, store it in a container.

Whenever you need to scrub your body, take 1 tablespoon as needed in the shower. Scrub your skin with the mixture and rinse well.

It will leave your skin smooth and silky.

Simple Salt Scrub

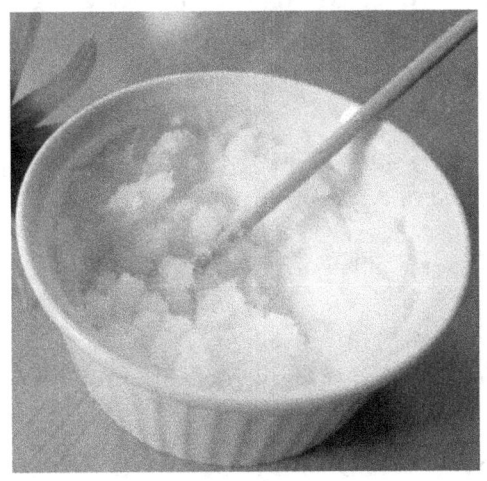

Ingredients required

1/2 cup almond oil

1 cup sea salt

15 drop high quality essential oils.

Preparation:

Take a small bowl and add salt to it.

Add the oil, and mix it well with a spoon. The texture should be moist enough to hold together.

Gently add the drops of essential oil and mix it well.

Your scrub is ready, store it in a container.

Whenever you need to scrub your body, just take 1 tablespoon as needed in the shower. Scrub your skin with the mixture and rinse well.

It will leave your skin smooth and silky.

Spa Sea Salt Scrub

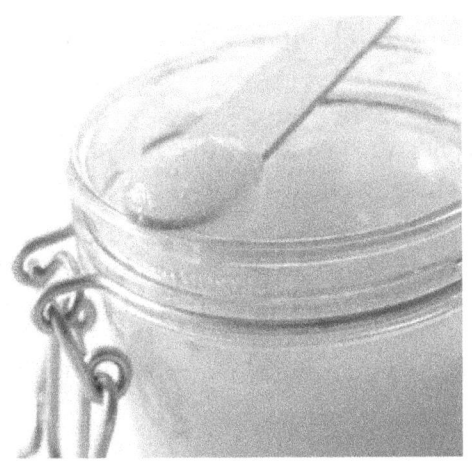

Ingredients required

2 cups sea salt

1 1/3 cups aloe Vera oil

2 tsp vitamin E oil

2 tablespoons honey

Instructions

Take a bowl and Combine all the ingredients except vitamin E oil.

Add Vitamin E oil into the mixture and mix it well.

Your scrub is ready; store it in an air tight container.

Add a bit to your hand or a bath mitt and rub all over and rinse off well.

It will leave your skin smooth and silky.

Olive Oil Salt Scrub

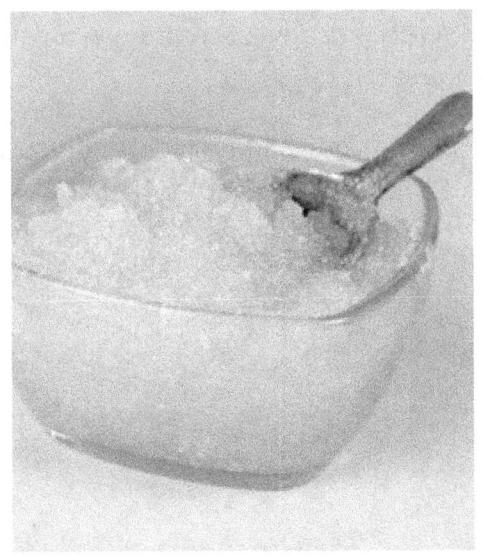

Ingredients required

1 tsp of Sea salt

1 tsp olive oil

Instructions

In a bowl mix equal amount of olive oil and salt. Let the salt soak up the oil.

Your scrub is ready; store it in an air tight container.

Add a bit to your hand or a bath mitt and rub all over and rinse off well.

It will leave your skin smooth and silky.

Baby Oil Sea Salt Scrub

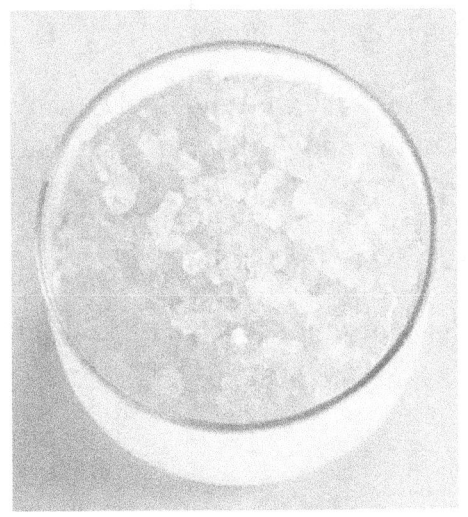

Ingredients required

1 cup sea salt

½ cup baby oil

Instructions

In a bowl mix well sea salt and baby oil.

Scrub is ready, store it into a screw top jar and leave it for 24 hours.

Stir the mixture well and apply to any areas of the body you wish to exfoliate.

Massage into the skin for a few minutes then shower off.

It will leave your skin smooth and silky.

Lavender Sea Salt Scrub

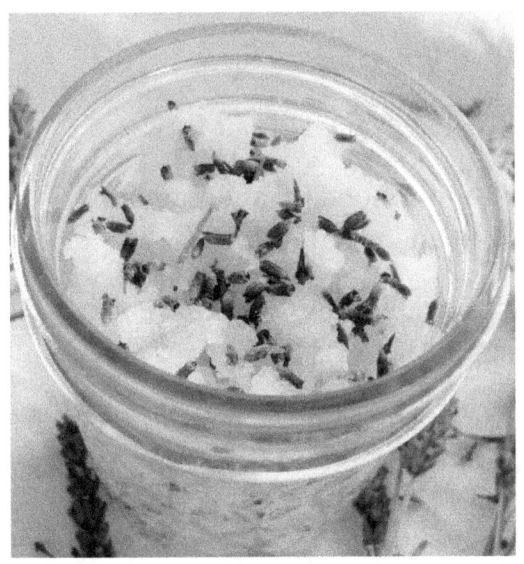

Ingredients:

1/2 cup sea salt

1/3 cup almond oil

2 tsp Vitamin E oil

1 tsp dried lavender

8 drops lavender oil

Instructions:

Take a bowl and add salt to it.

Now add almond Oil and Vitamin E oil to the salt and mix it well.

Add lavender flowers and lavender essential oil to salt and oil mixture.

Cover the mixture and let it sit for an hour.

Apply to dry or damp skin, massaging in circular motion.

Rinse with cool water in shower or bath.

It will leave your skin smooth and silky.

Rosemary Sea Salt Scrub

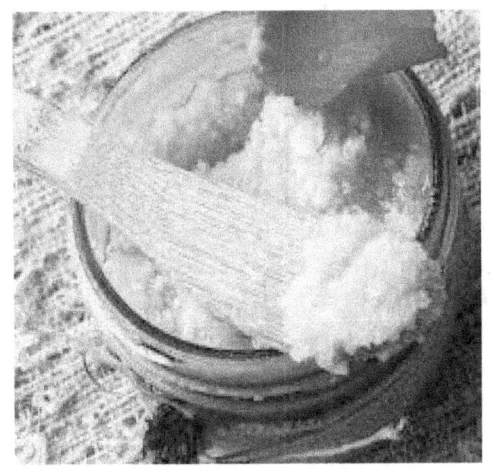

Ingredients:

2 cups sea salt

1 cup Olive Oil

1/4 oz. Liquid glycerin soap

5-10 Drops Rosemary essential oil

Instructions:

In a boiler take oil and soap and heat them.

Then stir in the salt and add the rosemary essential oils to it.

Let it cool down for some time.

Apply to dry or damp skin, massaging in circular motion.

Rinse with cool water in shower or bath.

It will leave your skin smooth and silky.

Citrus Salt Body Scrub

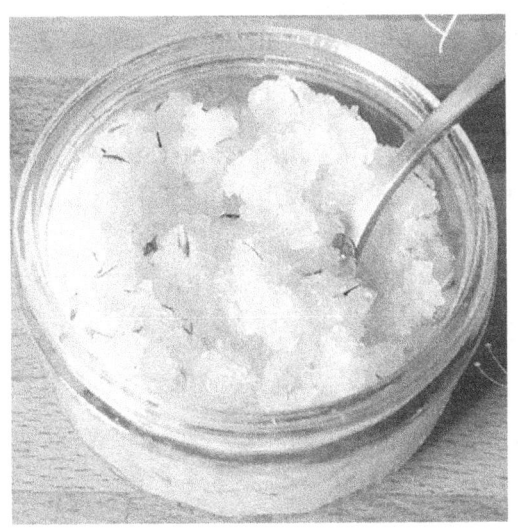

Ingredients:

1/2 cup sea salt

1/2 cup almond oil

1/2 tsp lemon zest

1/2 tsp orange zest

Instructions:

Take a bowl and add the ingredients to it except oil and mix them well.

Now gradually add almond oil to it, such that it forms a thick paste.

Pour the mixture into an airtight container and store in a cool dry place.

Apply to dry or damp skin, massaging in circular motion.

Rinse with cool water in shower or bath.

It will leave your skin smooth and silky.

Honey Salt Scrub

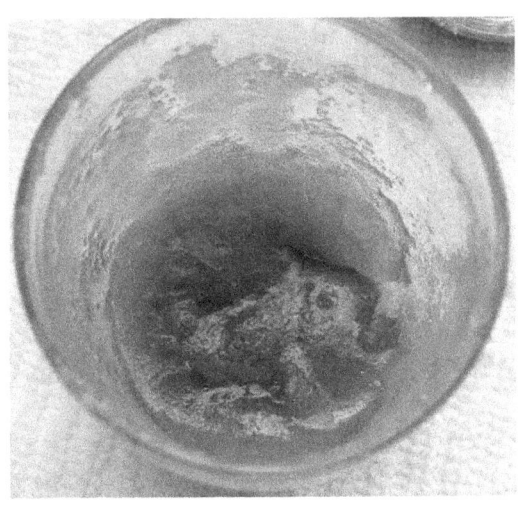

Ingredients required

1 cup Sea salt

1/2 cup almond or coconut Oil

5 - 15 drops Essential Oil

1 tbsp of honey

Instructions:

Mix all the ingredients except essential oil in a bowl.

Now gradually add essential oil as per the requirement to make a paste.

Your scrub is ready; store it in a tight container.

Massage gently into skin, and then rinse off with warm water.

It will leave your skin smooth and silky.

Rose Salt Scrub

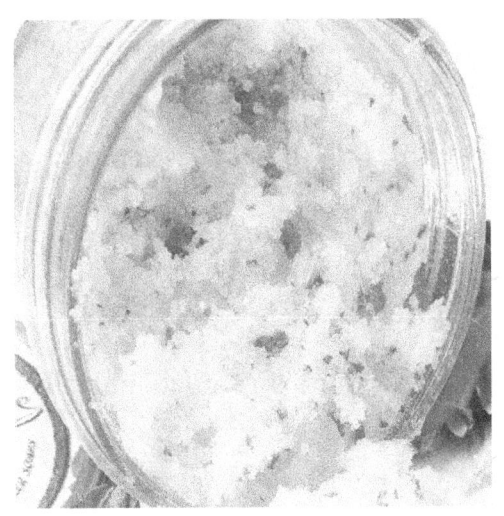

Ingredients required

1 cup Sea salt

1/2 cup almond or coconut Oil

5 - 15 drops Essential Oil

1 tbsp rose petals

Instructions:

Mix all the ingredients except essential oil in a bowl. Stir them well.

Now gradually add essential oil as per the requirement to make a paste.

Your scrub is ready; store it in a tight container.

Massage gently into skin, and then rinse off with warm water.

It will leave your skin smooth and silky.

<u>Lemon Salt Scrub</u>

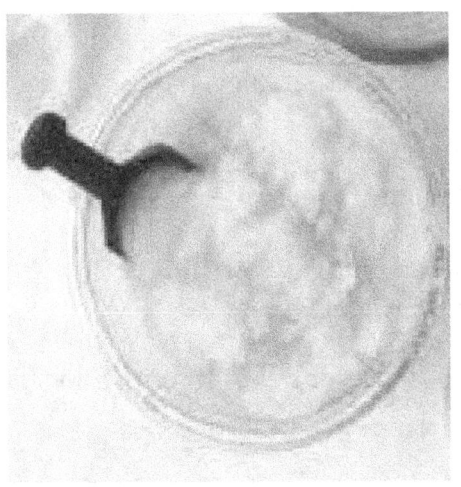

Ingredients required

1 cup Sea salt

1/2 cup almond or coconut Oil

5 - 15 drops Essential Oil

1/2 tsp of lemon

Instructions:

Mix all the ingredients except essential oil in a bowl. Stir them well.

Now gradually add essential oil as per the requirement to make a paste.

Your scrub is read; store it in a tight container.

Massage gently into skin, and then rinse off with warm water.

It will leave your skin smooth and silky.

Other Scrub Recipes

<u>Oatmeal Body Scrub</u>

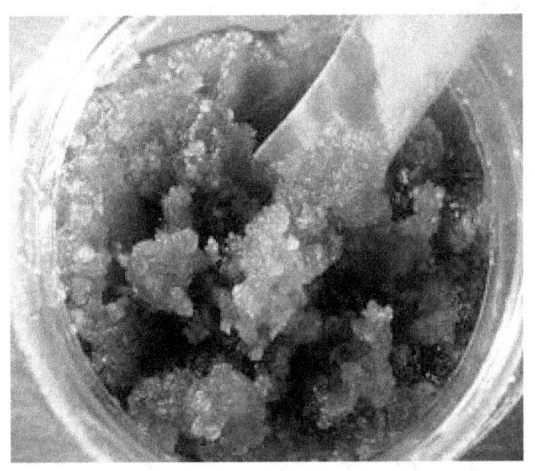

Ingredients:

1 cup oatmeal

8-10 drops of lavender essential oil

8-10 drops of tangerine

8-10 drops of rosewood

4-5 drops of chamomile

1 Tbsp dried lavender petals

Instructions:

Take a bowl and mix all the ingredients to it except the oils. Stir them well.

Now add essential oils drop by drop, stirring constantly to avoid clumps.

Scrub is ready; store it in an airtight jar in the fridge.

Massage gently into skin, and then rinse off with warm water.

It will leave your skin smooth and silky.

<u>Coffee Body Scrub</u>

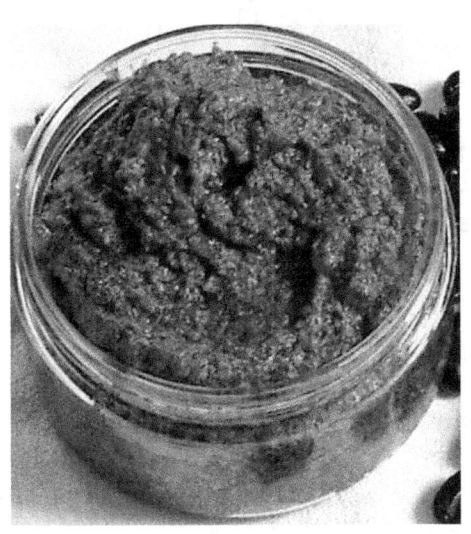

Ingredient Required

1 cup coffee

1 Tbsp salt

1/3 cup almond oil

1 tsp ground cinnamon

8-10 drops grapefruit essential oil

8-10 drops orange

4-4 drops peppermint

Instructions:

Take a bowl and mix all the ingredients to it except the oils. Stir them well.

Now add almond oil and grapefruit essential oils drop by drop, stirring constantly to avoid clumps.

Scrub is ready; store it in an airtight jar in the fridge.

Massage gently into skin, and then rinse off with warm water.

It will leave your skin smooth and silky.

Coffee Vanilla Scrub

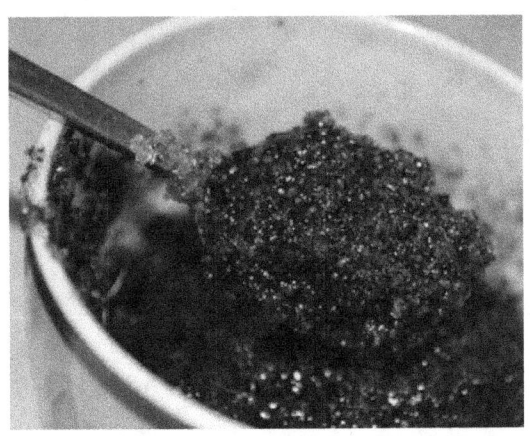

Ingredient Required

1 Cup Coffee

1 Cup Salt

1/2 Cup Coconut Oil

1/2 Tbsp Cinnamon

1 Tbsp Vanilla

Instructions:

Take a bowl and mix all the ingredients to it except the oils. Stir them well.

Now add coconut oil drop by drop, stirring constantly to avoid clumps.

Scrub is ready; store it in an airtight jar in the fridge.

Massage gently into skin, and then rinse off with warm water.

It will leave your skin smooth and silky.

<u>Oatmeal Chamomile Body Scrub</u>

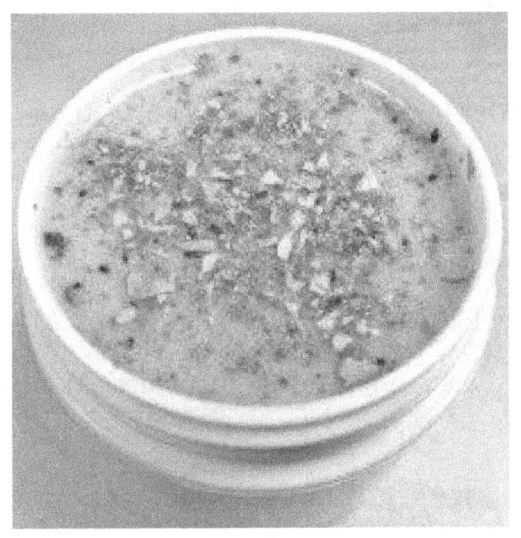

Ingredients required

1 cup oatmeal

1/2 cup coconut oil

1/2 cup grape seed oil

2 chamomile tea bags

Instructions

First take a grinder and grind the oats into dust form.

Take a bowl and mix all the ingredients to it except the oils. Stir them well.

Now add coconut oil and grape seed oil drop by drop, stirring constantly to avoid clumps.

Scrub is ready; store it in an airtight jar in the fridge.

Massage gently into skin, and then rinse off with warm water.

It will leave your skin smooth and silky.

These were some of the best and easy to make body scrubs at home. The best thing is that you can apply these scrubs on any part of your body and on your face as well. These are very effective and will add beauty to your face and looks.

Here are some facts and FAQ's on body scrubs:

Why You Should Use an Exfoliating Body Scrub?

We all want smooth and soft skin, especially in the summer time. And our body is covered in a layer of dead skin cells. The lotions that you apply on your skin works to keep your skin soft, but they don't work for so long. Dead skin cells still remain there. If you want healthy, smooth skin, there is no better way that using a body exfoliating (scrub). Take body scrub and rub it all over your body in a circular motion and rinse off. Make sure you moisturize immediately after you dry off. You'll instantly see the difference in your skin. It will appear younger and feel much softer.

What Skin Care Problems Does Exfoliation Help to Improve?

Exfoliation cures us from many skin problems. It destroys acne-causing bacteria; it also helps remove red, dark marks that remain on the skin long. Exfoliation is beneficial for breaking up the pigmented cells to allow them to fade. Combined with a skin lightening agent, such as Vitamin C, exfoliation will help accelerate the fading process. Especially in the winter, exfoliation is very important because in winter we have dry skin, so we tend to load up on heavier creams. And the more you layer on the heavier creams, the more you are trying to re-hydrate dry skin cells, which make no sense! Instead, increase your exfoliation to remove the dry skin cells, and then moisturize the new skin cells, resulting in a moister skin.

How Does A Person Know If They Are Getting Too Much Exfoliation?

If while using scrubs, your skin turns bright red and feels irritated afterwards, it means that the grains used in the scrub are too large. So at that time it is suggested to use the exfoliation once a week and it's good to consult with some skin specialist if you are using any chemical scrub.

What are the best essential oils for body scrub?

The best essential oils used in making homemade body scrubs are vanilla essential oil, camphor essential oil, cardamom essential oil, carrot essential oil, ginger essential oil, grapefruit essential oil, jasmine essential oil, lavender essential oil, lemon essential oil, orange essential oil, peppermint essential oil, etc.

Disadvantages of body scrub?

There really aren't any disadvantages of body scrubs, unless your body reacts poorly to it. Use it and see how your skin reacts. If you get a bad reaction just stop using it, else use it frequently once or twice a week and you will be benefitted from it.

NOTE

Try these body scrubs at your home and share your views with me. I hope you enjoyed reading the book and you will be benefitted from the book. Thanks for purchasing the book.

DISCLAIMER

This book is written with an intention to provide informative and useful material. It is not designed to treat, diagnose, prevent or cure any specific health condition or problem, nor is it intentional to replace the physician's advice. No action is advised to take solely on the contents. Before getting inferences and following any suggestions in this publication, readers are advised to consult their healthcare professional or physician first, on anything related to their health.

The publisher and author shall not be liable for any risk or loss, liability, personal or anything, as a consequence, openly or indirectly, from the use of any contents of this publication. All or any product names within this publication are the brands of their owners. None of them have authorized, sponsored, approved or endorsed this publication. Before using any of their products, always read all the information given on the product level. The publisher and author are not liable for any claim from the manufacturers.

Book 2

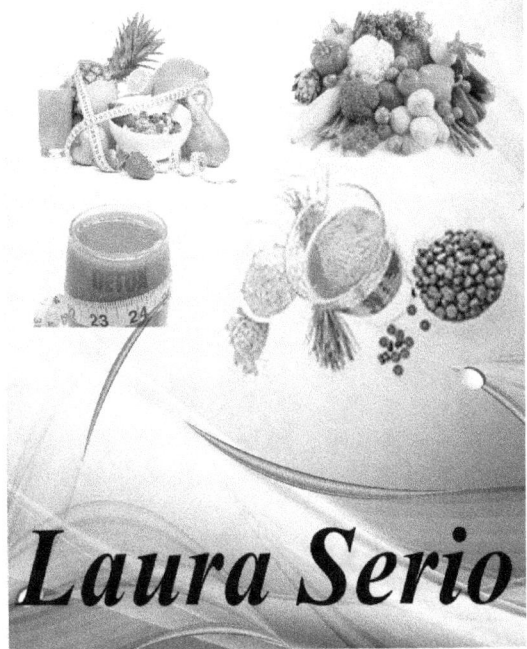

NATURAL BODY DETOX

How To Naturally Cleanse And Detox Your Body

Laura Serio

Natural Body Detox

How To Naturally Cleanse And Detox Your Body

By

Laura Serio

Natural Body Scrubs At Home

ACKNOWLEDGMENTS

For my students and friends, who all selflessly helped me in writing this book. Special thanks to those who asked, insisted and assisted me in turning the seminars in this practical form. All Rights Reserved 2012-2015 @ Laura Serio.

Table of Contents

INTRODUCTION

The focus of this book is to assist in the decision-making process involved with detoxification. This book should not be used in place of professional medical advice. My aim is to inform the reader of some points to consider when wanting to explore a detoxification regime. Those points include benefits and possible consequences, and proper reasoning to detoxify. Here in this book, I also mentioned the benefits of juicing, one of the easiest ways to detox. I do not recommend anyone to start a detox regime without consulting their health professional or doctor so as to ensure medications that they may be prescribed are not affected adversely.

CHAPTER 1
Myths About Detox

Detox is one of those very decisive topics. It seems that there is no clear majority on whether it is a positive or a negative. Speaking as one who was anti-detox before writing this book, in researching the topic enough positive evidence presented to open my eyes to the benefits. For those who are firmly against detox or haven't had any run-ins with detox, we are often filled with negative thoughts. "My body will take care of the toxins on its own," "Detoxifying is just another crazy Hollywood fad", or "I have heard that a detox regime will destroy my metabolism." But like everything that involves our health, good advice is often met with resistance. Let's take a closer look at each of these myths and see if we can get to the heart of the issue.

My Body Will Take Care Of The Toxins On Its Own

If this is a thought that has ever crossed your mind, take some time to think about it. Our body is an extremely complex organism that is built to extract what it needs from food and discard the rest. It has an intricate system that it uses to remove harmful waste and toxins. While there are steps our body takes to rid itself of toxins, it is not a 'get out of jail free card'.

It is ludicrous to think that our body on its own get rid us of all the toxins, especially in a day and age of preservatives. Our bodies are clearly not invincible. Years and years of unhealthy diet habits, poor exercise, and even the amount of sleep we get play a pivotal role in our body's ability to cleanse itself. When we don't get enough sleep, our bodies crave more sweets than we probably should. When we overdose on sweets, we don't get enough nutrients in our diet. All three, diet, exercise and sleep exists in a delicate balance.

Our body's natural detoxification system is somewhat like a filter for a fish tank. When the filter is brand new, we can clearly see it at work, cleaning the water. As time passes though, we begin to notice that the water is not coming out as clean as it was when we first got it. It is at this time that we begin to think about ways to help the filter to clean the water. The same is true for our body's natural filter as well. The filter has buildup on it prohibiting it from doing its job properly, it needs to be cleaned. So simply put doing a detox plan is like cleaning of the filter.

Detoxifying Is Just A Hollywood Fad

With celebrities such as Oprah, Donna Karen, Salma Hayek, and Demi Moore writing rave reviews, it is not easy to debunk this myth. I don't like to classify this as a myth, more as an excuse. If Hollywood stars have been using detox for years and we have seen the results on both the small and the big screens, what evidence are we seeing that this isn't true? We just have to sift through all the negative and positive feedback.

Though it does meet all of the requirements to be considered a fad, some of the regimes recommended by stars actually hold some weight. Beyoncé used a regime to lose 20 pounds for her 2006 role in 'Dreamgirls'. Salma Hayek uses a 3 day juice regime to give her skin a 'glow'.

It is probably a safe assumption to say there is something to these regimes. One must be cautious and conscientious when choosing their detox, as our bodies are not all the same. What works wonders for one person is not necessarily going to work for another. On the contrary, they can be quite catastrophic. Many stars agree that natural detox is the best way to go. It's all about what works for you. Just do your homework and put your common sense to work. Research and review until you find a detox regime that appeals to you, and then go right into it before committing yourself.

Will A Detox Regime Destroy My Metabolism?

This is a popular concern when it comes to the topic of detox. There is no medical evidence that states that a detox regime will have direct detrimental effects on metabolism, it all depends on the regimen. Here trouble arises, when we try to go on an extended fast without taking in the proper nutrients. A good rule of thumb is that if you're feeling hunger, it means that you're not getting the proper nutrients that your body needs. Many detox plans will call for eating exclusively one food group, or excluding a food group all together. Doing so can cause a body to run harmfully low on the nutrients it receives.

There your metabolism may end up getting negatively affected lies in taking part in an extended fast. Our bodies are not designed to go even 24 hours without water, and no more than a week to 10 days without food. Whenever you go more than 24-48 hours without eating, you run the risk of sending your body into a hibernation mode of sorts. When your body goes into hibernation mode, it slows down as your metabolism is brought to a much lower rate and your body shifts into a calorie conserving setting. Having this happen can cause some serious detrimental effects on your health. Permanent muscle loss, weakened immune system, low energy, irritability and even extreme mood swings are among those effects.

There are safe ways that people can fast though, that will be covered in the section "**Fasting as a spiritual exercise**".

Chapter 2
Spring Cleansing –
Detoxifying Your Body
Naturally

What Is Detoxifying?

Detoxifying is defined as: to remove a harmful substance (such as a poison or toxin) or its effects from a human body. This is pretty much self-explanatory. It is the process by which the liver, kidneys, and colon attempt to remove buildup in our bodies in order to make us feel better and have better health. As harsh as this word may sound at first, the actual process itself can be quite simple.

Some actually find detoxifying to be an enjoyable experience. This of course depends on the way in which you choose to go about it. Again, it's all about what works for YOU.

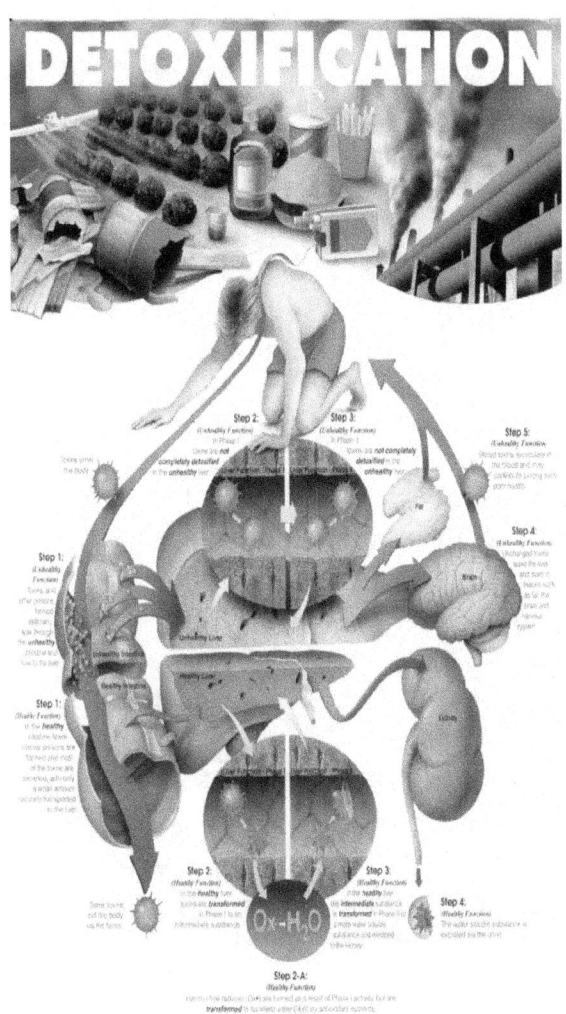

How Detoxifying Works

Detoxifying works in a variety of ways and can differ depending on the specific plan that you choose. In reality, they are just different ways to reach the desired results of being healthier. Make sure that you exercise caution in your selection, as not all detox plans are built equal. In a nutshell, they work by cutting out the things that are causing the toxic buildup, but in some cases, they also remove necessary items from the body, so you should be careful which system you choose. In essence, detoxing is an attempt to hit the reset button on the body's natural system for the removal of toxins.

What Is The Best Way To Detox?

Whenever the question arises of which detoxifying plan is the best, I always find myself grinning. The reason is that there is no one size fits all when it comes to detox. Just as with any health concern, a person's body, diet, and level of activity have a role to play in the effectiveness of the selected detox plan. Obviously, an all juice regimen is probably not at all a good idea for a world-class athlete or an all meat diet for a vegan. The less supplements and pills that are a required for the regime, the better it is. We are a complex organism living in a complex world, so there is no need to make detox more complex than it has to be. The best way to detox is to find a plan that still allows for the intake of proteins and nutrients. These are the building blocks of life. I cannot fathom how a regime can boost your health while prohibiting these.

The best way to detox is to rest the body, both food wise and lifestyle wise and to drink plenty of water. Our bodies are made almost all of water, so anything that returns the usual level of hydration is going to be good for us, unless, of course we have a condition, which prevents us from drinking as much water as we should. The lack of taste of water is not one of those conditions! The kidneys actually shrink, if they are not fully hydrated for a long period of time, so just keeping them in condition is going to be a positive.

But seriously, the best way to detox is to embark on a program that will only involve several hours. If you find this has helped, or you enjoyed it, then you can always expand the length next time.

What Are The Benefits Of Detoxifying?

There are many benefits to detoxifying. In this section, I'll introduce its benefits and give the why behind it.

Energy boost - This is a common claim by practitioners of all different sorts of detox plans. As our bodies remove caffeine, saturated fats, trans fats, and sugars, we find that our bodies feel less 'weighed down' giving us a feeling of energy. Also by eating more produce, we take advantage of a natural source of energy that will not result in a 'crash'. A detox plan actually helps your body to be more readily able to tap this energy source.

Many would credit a cut in caloric intake or as the reason behind dramatic weight loss. However, if you make the conscience effort to rid yourself of bad habits, and exercise regularly, you will find that weight loss from a quick detox can be sustainable. After all, if you are just looking to shed some weight for only a few days, I am sure you would like to keep it off for the remaining of your days.

Giving the body a rest - This is very important to do. We continually bombard our systems with the wrong types of food and fluids. Taking a day away from this pattern gives the inner body a chance to really eliminate old remnants of food and other toxins from the body without stressing out over more being dumped on it.

Liver cleansing - The liver is the main inner body organ, which works its butt off to rid you of toxins. Sometimes, it can get overwhelmed by our thoughtlessness on what we eat and drink. Giving it a fasting juice day will help it to re-regulate itself and restart producing clean useful bile, which also helps with weight loss, instead of sticky stuff that the bile ducts cannot squeeze outwhen it is needed.

Detoxing can also aid in the spiritual development of a person. When the body is not focusing on metabolizing food, it is free to wander at will. Many spiritual guides speak of the cleansing effect detoxing has on their upper minds too.

CHAPTER 3
Rejuvenate, Recharge, And Renew Your Body

Get In Shape While Getting Rid Of Toxins

We are all guilty of saying we need to get in shape. Whenever we look through yearbooks, ponder over former athletic feats, or think about the good old days when you could get up a flight of stairs without at least breathing a little heavier; these are probably the times, we most want to return our bodies to its former glory. That's where it ends for most people, with wishing they could return to these days. Such people might go drop $100-$200 on fancy gear, gym memberships, and protein bars or shakes. They might throw away a fridge full of junk food and replenish it with healthy everything. Then the actual work comes in - The dreaded sweating, panting, overheating. By the time a couple days have passed, around 90% of people have thrown in the towel.

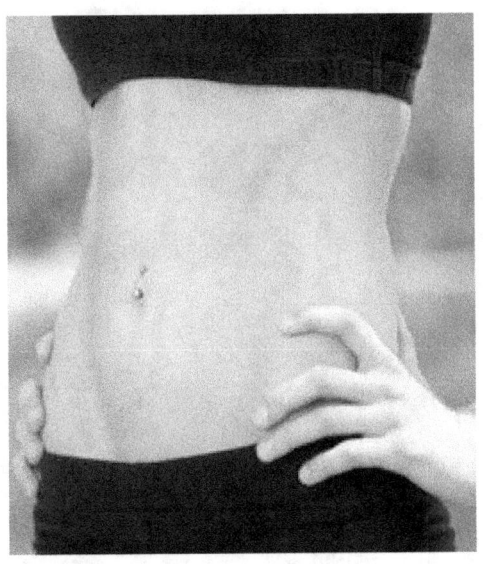

When thinking about it from a detoxification standpoint, think about all the negative effects that toxins are having on your body. After the first couple days of exercising, you should begin to see the benefits of proper nutrition and your new active lifestyle. Stick with it - The benefits will begin to intensify. You're giving those toxins an extra avenue to leave your body through pores when you sweat. So, greatly accelerate the detoxification process. It creates a cycle that will make your goal far more achievable.

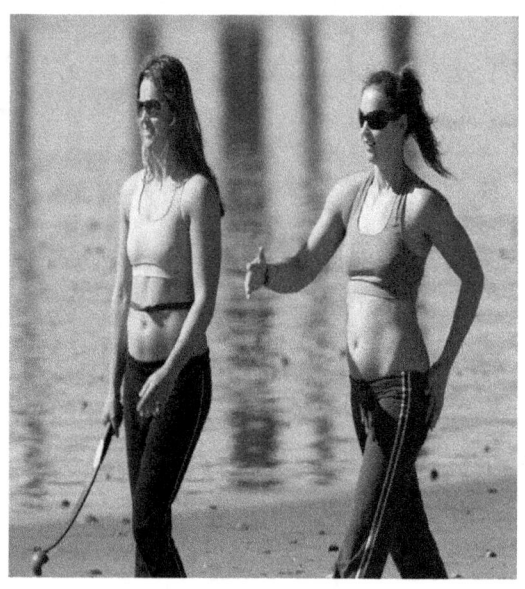

Exercise is not hard work to be useful to detoxing, but it does have to be regular and continuous. A 5-minute walk around the yard every day will do more good in the long run than simply doing nothing at all. But combining a detoxing day and exercise should be viewed with caution. Your body is accustomed to being full of food or fluid. If you have started on a juicing routine, then allow yourself some time to understand how you feel before throwing yourself into a heavy exercise routine. You do not want to fall flat on your face from unexpected results coming from your body's reaction to the juicing routine. Slow, steady, and be aware of any adverse reactions.

Active Lifestyle

If there is only one point you take away from this book, let it be the importance of maintaining an active lifestyle. There are so many benefits to it; I could write a book on the benefits of getting up, getting out, and getting your exercise. As with everything health (and New Year's resolutions!) related, the beginning days are a very crucial period.

After the adrenaline from the excitement about deciding to get in shape wears off, we begin to feel sluggish or overwhelmed and don't think we can carry on. I'm not gonna lie and say it'll be easy. However, this next nugget may be some motivation. By exercising our body will actually become an energy creating machine! With all that extra energy, you'll have plenty to feed your active lifestyle.

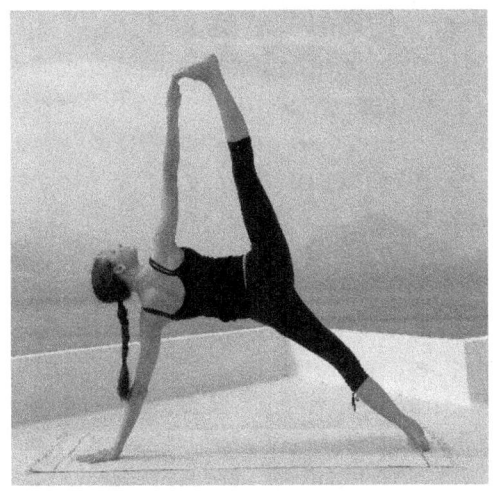

We all know that it requires energy to do exercise, but how many knew that doing exercise can actually increase your energy production? So by exercising not only do we find a way to give ourselves more energy, but we also help to speed the detoxification process. Can you see how exercise creates a beneficial cycle for our bodies?

This is not all that exercise will do for you. It will increase the body's blood circulation, which helps nutrient transportation to the muscles and tissue.

Simultaneously lymph fluids circulate through the body collecting up all the toxic grime from our body's cells. These fluids are secreted at a much higher level when we exercise properly. Remember, if you're not sweating you're not exercising properly.

I am sorry to burst your bubble if you consider sweating is simply an unpleasant experience and does not need to be undergone. Sweat is very necessary to remove toxins. It also helps to regulate our temperature. If we do not sweat, we may end up being too hot internally and that is equally as bad for us as being too cold.

Meals

Depending on the detox plan that you choose, your meals may seriously restricted. Let this be a huge factor in which detox plan you participate in. Make sure that your body is getting all the proper nutrients that it requires. Vitamins and nutrient pills may be something worth considering, but, as these are artificial, you need not to go that way.

There are foods such as radishes that have super food qualities, which are jam-packed with all those little technical things our body is built upon. A little research will show you which vegetables and fruit will give the most vitamins and nutrients when used in juicing detoxes. Or you can research different colors and their benefits as some colors have more of antioxidants than either minerals or vitamins.

What Am I Going To Eat?

Kiwi fruit is another such super food as it ranks near the top of the list as far as nutritionally packed fruits go. It is also one of the few fruits that contain vitamin E, which most Americans do not get enough of. The kiwi fruit is a great fruit to use in your juicer, if you make the decision that a juice fast would be the best form of a detox plan for you.

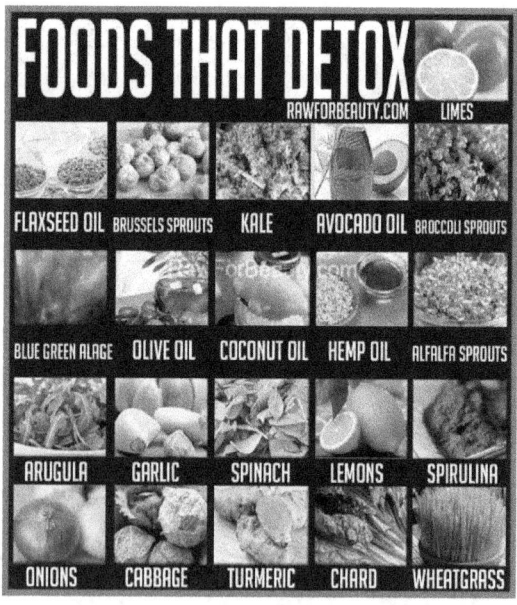

Nuts is a well known healthy food that has taken a beating because of the high fat content. However, in small doses they are a great way to get protein in. If you join a detox plan, check what they allow in your diet. But it's a great way to keep your health on track afterwards... as long as you watch your portions. Portion sizes of anything are worth another book, so go for the recommended ones in a health and nutrition book.

You should not simply leave out or include certain things just because some star says they do so. I have seen some diets that consist simply of food that has no use apart from conning the body into thinking it has been fed for a short while, only to realize the con and slam the person with an almighty attack of the munchies! These stars usually have coping mechanisms to deal with this result, which ordinary people do not have, but do not mention them!

Choose juices and plenty of water. These will give your body necessary fluids. The body can survive a

135

surprisingly long amount of time without food, but finds itself in a lot of trouble very quickly without fluids. Heavy fluids such as milk can be avoided as they may encourage a bout of diarrhea because there is nothing else in the stomach. Coffee is also not recommended - after all, you are trying to get rid of toxins!

Are detox diets really worth doing?

Whether or not a detox diet is really worth doing depends on what it is that you seek to accomplish from the experience. If your reasons for seeking to start a detox plan are spiritually motivated then by all means go for it. Just make sure that you know exactly what it is you are trying to do and that you have consulted your higher power. There are times in life when we feel that our higher power asks us to show a level of devotion, and this can be a quite spiritual experience.

Monks and other spiritual people often fast for several days, but their bodies are usually accustomed to this. The ordinary person is not, so a fasting period more than 2 days will have negative effects on them. Be sensible, especially if this is your first foray into this experience. This is also where juicing can assist with unexpected side effects.

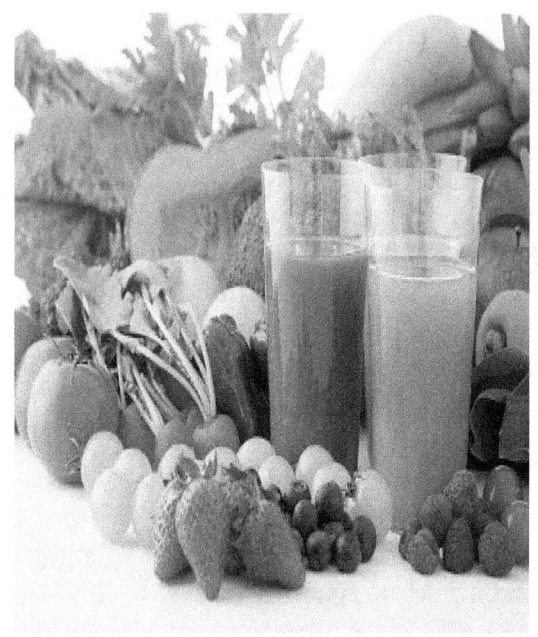

Another good reason for undertaking a detoxifying would be to clean out your body of all the debilitating poisons in an effort to begin a healthier lifestyle. A detox plan is not designed to be a counterweight to all the unhealthy habits that caused for the toxic buildup in the first place. When detoxes are properly utilized, they are a great decision.

With all the research I have collected, it becomes clear to me that doing a detox plan or any type of a fast for weight loss alone can be a bad decision. Statistics show that most people who lose weight while on a detox plan often have the weight return within a few days after the fast/detox is over. There are two major reasons for this.

Firstly, most of the initial weight loss comes from water weight. The second being that as soon as the detox is over most people go right back to the health habits that caused them to seek a weight loss solution in the first place. So if you're not really committed to making the necessary alterations to your diet and exercise schedule after the detox is over, then I would suggest you save your time and effort and just forget about detoxifying. In this case, you'll be playing Russian roulette with your health for a few short-lived benefits.

In order not to go straight back to your previous lifestyle before the detox or juicing regime, you should have a follow-up plan to use designed to take straight over. Perhaps reintroduce things one at a time to see what effect they have if you have had problems with gluten for instance. Or resolve to continue the juicing program for longer. There are many ways you can continue the benefits of detoxing - you do not have to stick strictly to the regime still.

CHAPTER 4
Detoxifying While Keeping Up With Everyday Demands

Our lives are very busy and demanding between school, work, and maybe religion, raising a family and trying to come up with enough sleep. Taking the time to make sure that we properly detoxify our system can be a daunting task. But doing so is not as hard as people believe that it is. It just takes some planning and discipline.

Home workers

Homeworkers get the edge when it comes to the diet and nutrition side of detoxifying, not to take away from their work. Their jobs are jobs nonetheless. But when you only have to answer to yourself as to how you organize your detox regime for the day, and then make the most of it! Ideally, choose a day when you do not have a million and one things already lined up. This will make it easier to stick to your plan.

One advantage or disadvantage of detoxes is that they can and do make some people very sleepy. If you feel this way, put yourself to bed and have a nap. The extra sleep time will also have positive effects on you. Leave your next item in the detox plan or juicing routine ready for when you wake and carry on. You will have not interfered with anything important and you will have gained some benefits. Look on the extra nap as a 'nanny nap', which have become a key player in a lot of stress busting routines recently.

Multitasking has been seen as an advantage for a long time. Unfortunately, this is not true. Studies have shown if we concentrate on doing one thing at a time, then we will almost certainly finish it. So divide your time properly. If you work from home, then you organize your fasting materials or your juices first before starting work. This will also remove the temptation to snack as you work as your detox fluid or food and your juices are ready to be consumed. Just apply a little willpower!

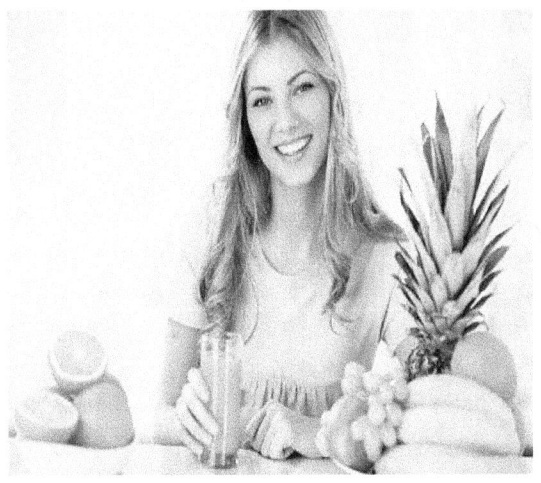

Whatever system you choose for detoxing your attention should be on it. Too many times, it is easy to have great intentions, only to be derailed by not having a plan in place. Most of us know it takes time and care to look after small children. If you have them in the house with you and you plan a detox day, you should refine your plan to either have something in place to occupy them fully so they are underfoot as little as possible.

Ideally, have a relative or friend take them for the day so you can concentrate on what you are doing and relax. This may sound selfish, but it is better than resenting the children for not allowing you to help yourself.

Detoxing is very good if it is the ONLY thing you are attempting to do for that day. Making meals is almost guaranteed to derail you, even if you only taste a tad of what you are cooking, so have food made up just for that day. Involve your family in what you are attempting, even if it is only telling them what you are trying.

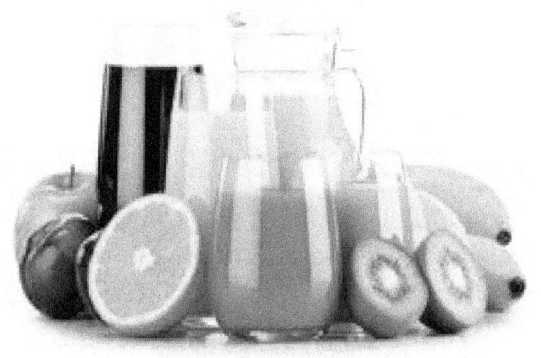

Stay At Home Parents

Though you may not want to throw your kids on a detox, you have a unique opportunity to monitor the amount of potential toxins your kid intakes through processed foods and all those 'extras' added to our foods these days. Choose a day when they have nothing much on and make it a fun exercise. Remember not to make it for any longer than 12 hours, or you will have more trouble than you wish. If you involve children in what you are doing, you often have a greater chance of it succeeding.

However, children's bodies react in different manner than an adult's body does to different things, so be careful about how much involvement in detoxification you do with your children. After all, it is not them you really need to detox, although you may think so!

Juicing on the other hand will introduce the child to fruits and vegetables that they may object to in whole foods and encourage them to drink them instead of eating them. Swap homemade juices for the glasses of cordial they are accustomed to at lunch or for a snack. Or make up healthy snacks with your juicer to take the place of a 'processed' food.

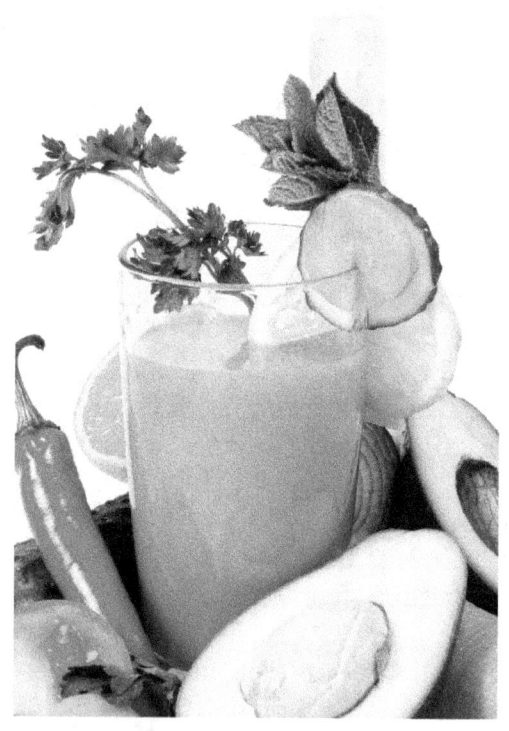

Pregnant/New Moms

Nutrition, did I mention nutrition. I don't wanna beat a dead horse, but nutrition! Nutrition is the idea of a detox diet, but if you've either just given birth to a baby or you have one growing inside of you, you should take care with drastic changes in your diet, even for one day. If you are not pregnant or a new mom, I apologize.

You have my permission to skip this section, although there are some pieces that apply to both pregnant and not pregnant women.

I'd like to share some tips of fasting for pregnant women. If properly planned and executed, a short fast can be pulled off in a breeze with no permanent health consequences. No long fast should be attempted at any time during a pregnancy. There are too many risks involved, for both fetus and mother.

Here are some tips to accomplish a very safe fast or detox program. Please remember that no fast, for any period of time, is a risk-free endeavor.

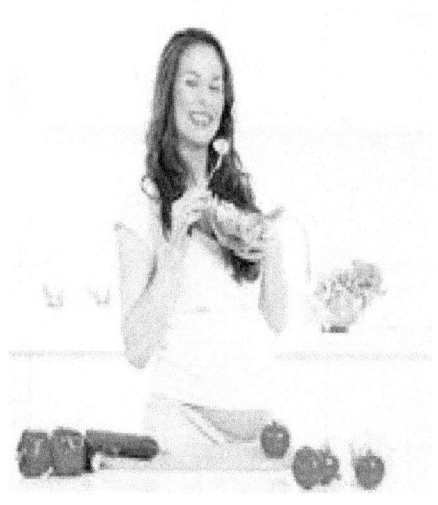

Make sure you discuss your fasting plans with your doctor or midwife before you even consider doing one or the other seriously. The below factors should be considered in depth:

- Is the detox or juicing regimen going to be healthy enough to be low risk to the pregnancy?
- What should I add to the detox or juicing regime to ensure the baby does not miss out on anything?

- Slow down as much as possible to lower stress on both baby and mother
- Do not consider a detox program or a juicing day if you suffer from any complications with your pregnancy such as pre-gestational diabetes, hypertension or anything else
- Use your common sense
- A juicing regime is not recommended if you are breastfeeding as the juice can come through in the milk and cause the baby discomfort or an upset bowel

Here are some of the signs you should abandon your fast:

- Bleeding (even light)
- Contractions 4 per hour
- Clear decrease in fetal movement
- Blurred vision
- Intense headache. This is not only for pregnant women. Get medical advice as soon as

possible if a headache od bad proportions develops

- Extreme weakness/fatigue. Also not only for pregnant women. All those who are on a detox routine should cease doing so immediately if they feel any of this. A sleepiness feeling is perfectly normal. Extreme anything is not.
- Dizziness. Moderate to severe lightheadedness. As above. Call for help if this happens because of the risk of falling and hurting yourself.

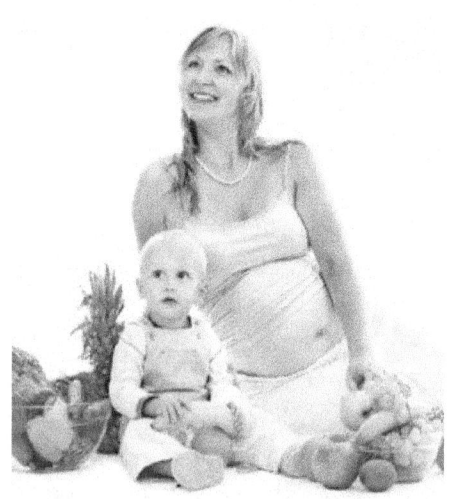

Chapter 5
The Spiritual Factors

Does A Clean Body Lead To A Clear Mind?

Many of the older artists and writers said that their mind worked better if they were hungry. This is possibly true, although the days of starving in a garret are long gone. Now we often are hungry, but it is not a lack of food that makes us that way. Rather it is a matter of too much unsuitable foods or a lack of healthy foods and fluids that is our problem. You can starve even while stuffing yourself, and this in turn reflects through our spiritual being.

When our body is free of toxins, our mind is in result freed. The best way that I can explain this is to explain the effects the toxins have. All those toxic agents that are not being excreted from your body take up space inside cells in the

151

body. When you remove those toxins, more space is made inside the cell for oxygen. Since each cell in your body can hold more oxygen, your heart has to do less work. When you get more oxygen your body can create more energy. The more energy you have, the better you feel. Couple with the fact that your heart has to work less, and you can see why it is that your mind clears up.

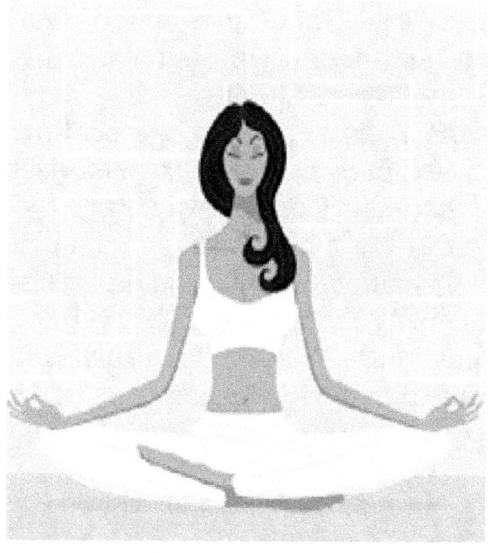

But just having a clearer mind is not the only benefit of having a clean body. As the gunk, junk, grime whatever you wish to call it is removed, you feel less 'weighed' down. Not being so congested, and having a clear head will make it much easier to control our emotions. Better control of your emotions will lead to less stress in your life. Your heart will thank you for taking pressure off it, as stress has been shown to narrow the vessels in spasm if the stress is very severe. This spasming is also felt all the way through all the vessels, so some damage has to occur if it is allowed to continue.

Fasting As A Spiritual Exercise

Fasting is one of the oldest forms of a spiritual journey in religions. It can be found in the Old Testament when Moses fasted for forty days in preparation for his meeting with the Lord on Mt. Sinai. Even Jesus, the central figure of Christianity, fasted in preparation for the ministry he would immediately take up after. This illustrates that fasting can be a way for one to go through a spiritual cleansing. If it can be used to spiritually cleanse us, wouldn't it make sense that it would help cleanse us in other ways.

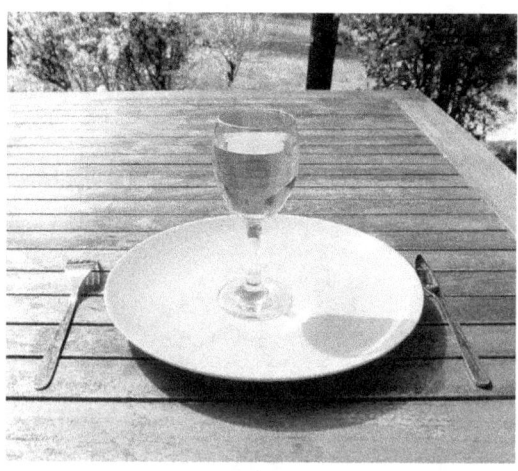

Many people have found that reading a book on spiritual activities such as the Qur'an or the Bible, even as just for reading purposes, combined with a detoxifying regime or juicing day makes them feel lighter and more relaxed in themselves. Answers to questions that have seemed impossible to resolve have been found. This is possible because of the body systems not requiring a great deal of energy to metabolize the food in them and so blood and nutrients are more available to the brain, but still... The thought that your higher self is better connected to you is very much in such people's minds.

No matter if, you consider yourself a spiritual person or not, you may gain more spiritual insight into yourself after a detox program or a juicing day than you ever had. That's an interesting thought, isn't it?

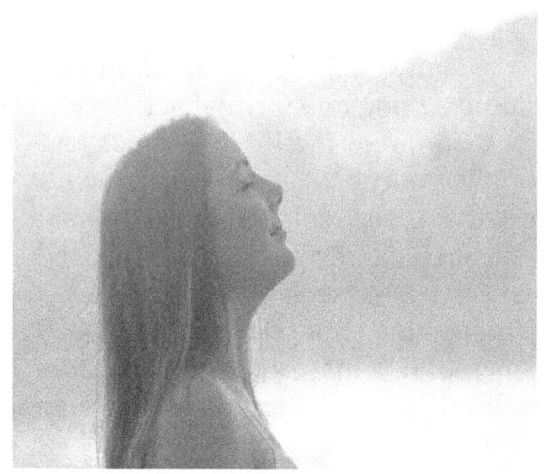

Spirituality is very much a personal thing to each and every one of us, and simple thought processes to some of us are a spiritual thing. So whatever can help us to think clearer and better is a help too.

Other Thoughts On Detoxifying

This book cannot cover all the ins and outs of detoxing or indeed even juicing as well as it should. To do that it would take around hundreds of chapters. All I am trying to do here is to give you a brief idea of what you can expect and why I think juicing or detoxing is worthwhile investigating from a health view.

I am NOT a medical professional, so I stress most seriously that you consult a health professional or your doctor before starting a fast or a major change to your diet. Not to do this can risk undoing all the good you are trying to do, especially if you are on prescribed medications. Some medications need proper food of some type to work or even to ensure they do not cause another problem. So do, please, consult your doctor BEFORE you start any change.

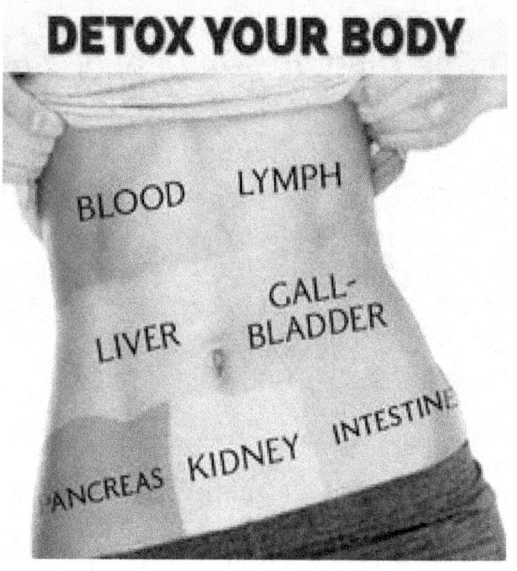

Detoxes and juicing will not work immediately. Nothing will. Anything that says you will lose X amount of weight in one day should be treated with disdain and be avoided like the plague. It always takes time to put the weight on, to become as unhealthy as you consider yourself nowadays or simply you have added ageing to your life. Detoxing or juicing is not going to cure everything or return you to the old you overnight. But, over time, either or will help you to feel better, both mentally and physically. The thought of being cleansed inside where it is not visible can have amazing effects on the outer side of us. Skin and eyes brighten and our outlook may improve by leaps and bounds. Even our other senses can be heightened.

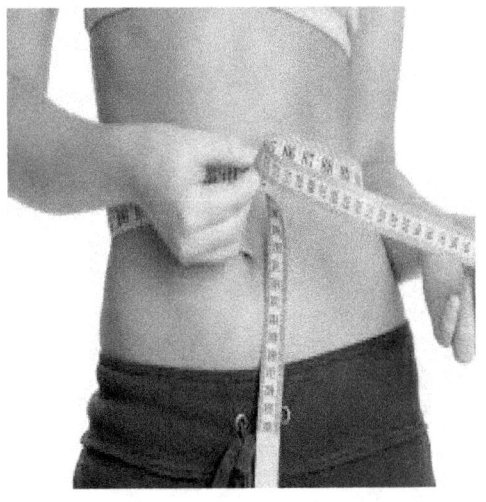

It also depends on your age. People who are reaching their outer stages of life will also benefit from detoxing or juicing, but the benefits they see will be entirely different to a person of 20 or 30. This is just something that goes with growing older and more mature. Our digestive systems and liver, however, are never too old to benefit from either detoxing or juicing days.

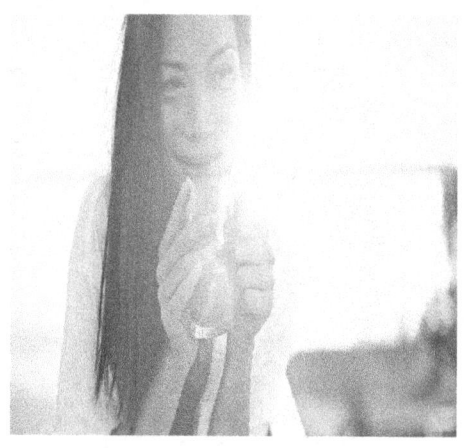

What Are Some Things I Should Avoid?

Caffeine is a drug. Of choice, of course, but still a drug and we have been quietly feeding our habit for hundreds of years. The thought of depriving ourselves of our favorite beverage of coffee is enough to bring many of us out in a cold sweat. This is a sure sign of addiction.

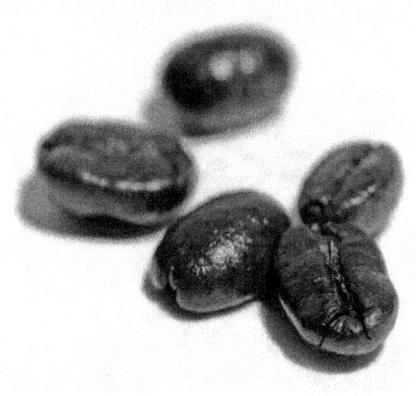

Unfortunately, the removal of caffeine from our daily life, if only for a day, is part of a detoxification program. We are detoxing after all, so we must remove ALL toxins. The removal of caffeine from the daily intake of fluids may bring a very unpleasant range of withdrawal symptoms, including nausea, severe headaches and bad mood swings. Try to focus on the benefits your body is getting by these symptoms as they will indicate that the caffeine level is being lowered. If necessary, go to bed and sleep. Drink plenty of water. These signs will go away. And when your detox or juicing day is finished, you may find you do not regard coffee or caffeine as the be-all and end-all that it once was.

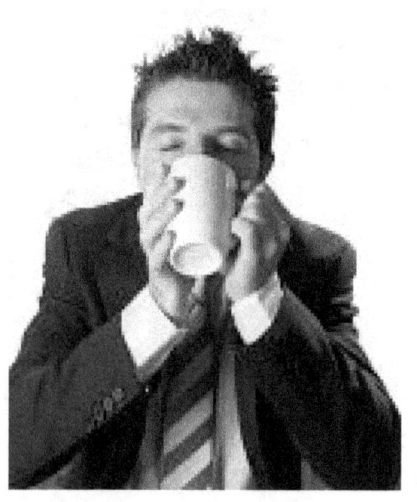

Empty calories. You can get them anywhere, from white bread to doughnuts and many ready-to-eat meals. These give you a quick hit of sugar and raise the level fast, but then allow you a downturn that encourages you to top up again quickly. Replace them with something else. Even chewing gum is better for you in terms of calories and the chewing motion fools your brain for a while that it is actually eating something solid.

Although exercise is certainly a help, starting a detox or juicing regime is not a signal to rush out and throw you into gym work or join marathon runners going on a 50-kilometer gallop. If that thought of starting an exercise regime plus detoxing or juicing frightens the daylights out of you, do NOT. You will only fail and make yourself miserable. Add a walk around your yard or to the corner of your street or something simple at first. As you gain confidence, extend yourself little by little. You may only go another house block each day. The thing is to have it as part of your ritual. There is plenty of time to add to your regime as you become fitter.

Along with your juicing or detox, drink plenty of water. As mentioned before, the kidneys can shrink over a long period of not being fully hydrated, and just because they extract toxins does not mean that they do not need hydrating themselves. A hydrated kidney can remove far more toxins quickly because it can function properly. So aim for a liter. Alternatively, whatever your doctor suggests per day to keep your kidneys working well.

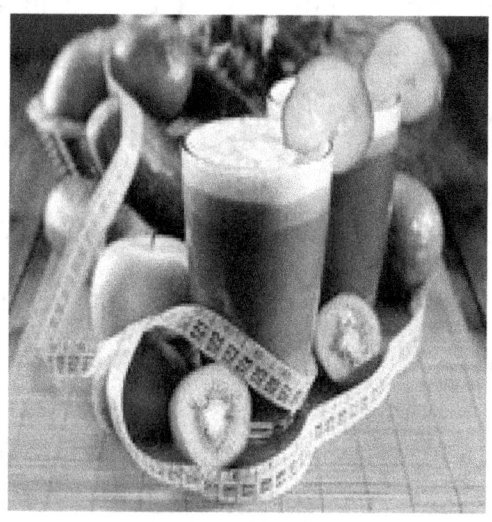

Experiment with herbs. Salt makes a lot of food very tasty indeed, but it is not good for us in large amounts. Try out different combinations of herbs and spices with your juices and detoxes and add less salt and sugar. Basil and tomato is a perfect example, or parsley and tomato and onion.

How That Translates To Detoxification

Reinforced positive thinking keeps up moral. A fast is a near to or complete withdrawal of food and or water. Or other stringent intake guidelines, which mean a period where there won't be those toxins in your system and your body, can catch up on waste removal. Jump starting the process of your body creating energy that is more natural.

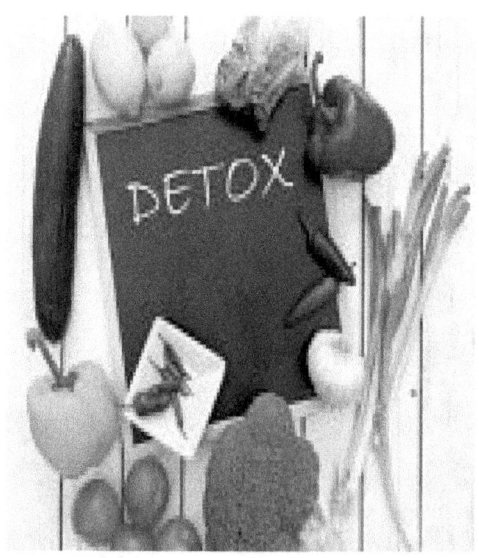

CHAPTER 6
Detoxifying Ingredients And Home Remedies

Ailments That Result From Toxins

Ailments, which are a direct result of toxins, are often self-inflicted. Who hasn't seen a play or a movie about old England when the gentleman has partaken of too much port and been forced to retire to his bed with a good dose of gout? Or the young rake who is suffering from one of his frequent binges with booze?

These ailments are only some of the damage that can occur when we overindulge in something pleasant, which can quickly turn against us. Among others, cancers, chemicals and autoimmune disorders are very prevalent and some which can have been avoided.

Detox As A Treatment

Heavy metal toxins are often removed by a series of detoxifying procedures with good results. Unfortunately, with heavy metals, the person may only discover they have been exposed when it is too late to do much good with any procedure apart from making the person comfortable. Asbestos poisoning is one of these, as it leads from very old paint. Juicing has been found to deliver much needed vitamins and minerals to these sufferers.

The treatment of these has not been found to be very successful, even though detoxification methods.

Detox is used with good results for drug addicts, though, once the drug is out of the person's system, the reason for the addiction has to be addressed, or the same old circle will start again. Alcohol and smoking are often also addressed using both juicing and detox. Getting nutrition into these people is the main aim at first, then whatever method is supplemented by counseling and perhaps the introduction of chemical compounds as a backup.

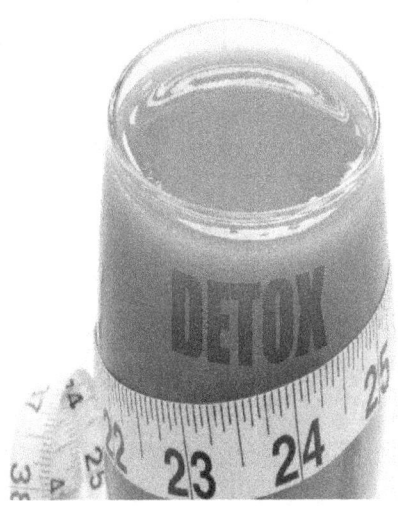

Detox As A Preventative Measure

Many stars of movies and music and even some authors book themselves into clinics at great expense to refresh themselves from their excesses. These excesses are often what normal people would consider every day, but, in the world that these people live in, looks are everything.

Days of very small meals, no alcohol, exercise and other things are practiced at health spas. Special seaweed wraps for the skin, maybe some plastic surgery, all of these are ways to detox. This can often turn into a double-edged sword if the participator goes back to the well too often, as there is only a limited amount of skin that can be stretched, twisted and shaped.

On nights when there is a large gathering, such as the Oscars, many of the people taking part will have undergone some type of detoxing for the night. It may be a day of juicing or a full week of some detoxing program, often designed by the person themselves so as not to show bloat, skin problems or to remove a few excess pounds.

Chapter 7
Juicing- Will It Help Detoxify?

Yes juicing will help your detoxification process. It allows for your body to be able to receive a compact dose of vitamins and nutrients without needing to take pills. Juicing is the new kid on the block where detoxifying is concerned, but savvy people have for years spent a day here and there drinking nothing but tea, or water in order to help their bodies, so it is not so new after all. Fruit juices have always been considered valuable as far as removing flatulence and bloat from the body, as well as kick starting the metabolism in the mornings by way of warm water and lemon juice. Added to these benefits, the loss of a few pounds has been the reason to have juice days.

Juicing is another string to the bow of detoxifying when you do not want to go fully into a detox regime lasting days. Juicing can be done over a day once a week and be used to regulate our eating habits. To add juicing to an already planned detox regime can be good thinking. The answer to this question is yes.

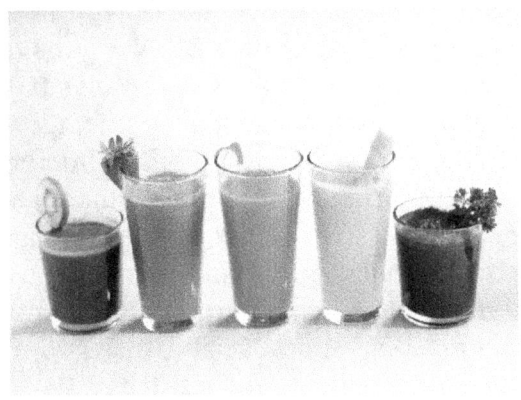

Myths/Facts

As with any treatment or procedure, myths abound everywhere. Some of these have been dealt with in the beginning of this eBook. Other myths are that detoxing can change a person's basic personality, not proven; that juicing will make a person refuse to eat solid food, again not proven; and the stomach will shrink. Unless the detox or the juicing is carried on far longer than it is stated to do so, then the stomach will start to lose some elasticity because it is accustomed to being stretched to full capacity.

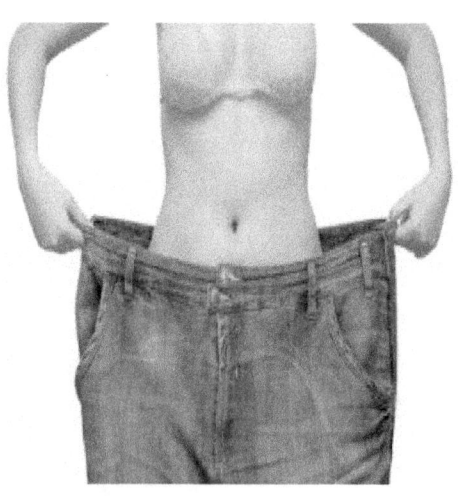

However, most of these are just that - myths. The facts are that detoxes and juicing days, done by following a good instruction video or book, will help you out with several problems, such as bloating and fluid retention. Like many things, detoxing and juicing days should be done on a regular basic but not every day.

Benefits

Juicing is one of the best ways to make sure that your body is still receiving proper nutrients while you are on a detox plan. It prevents your body from becoming malnutrition. As stated earlier malnutrition is the cause for most of the major side effects of a fast or improperly undertaken detoxification process. By using a detox plan that incorporates juicing, you reduce the risks you are taking dramatically.

Juicing, as claimed by Salma Hayek, can also help make your skin glow. It also makes it easier to get through a fast. Gives you a taste of something besides water and broth if you are on a wet fast. When using detox as a weight loss jump starter, it is recommended using juicing to replace one meal a day. This allows your body to receive most of the nutrients while cutting out a majority of the trans-fat and other unhealthy components in our meals. Making a sweet glass of juice can be an effective way to stave off chocolate and other junk food cravings.

How To Apply Juicing To Your Detox Process

A lot of the times, you will be able to find a detox process that already incorporates or depends entirely upon juicing to cut the work. One thing you do need to keep in mind when juicing is that most to all of the fiber from fruits and veggies are cut out when the juice is extracted from your ingredient. Now fiber plays a vital role in cleansing our colons. The fiber scrapes along the side of the colon as waste is passed through. By cutting out the fiber, you may be minimizing detoxification effects.

A good way to counteract this while keeping your juicing plan is to add a little of the pulp back into the juice. This keeps you guilt free. The pulp, while not as much fiber as the whole fruit or veggie. Many have complained of cases of diarrhea when doing a wet fast or a juice detox. A wet fast is where you consume no solid foods, but you do drink water, broth, and/or some juices. A wet fast is much healthier in comparison to a dry fast.

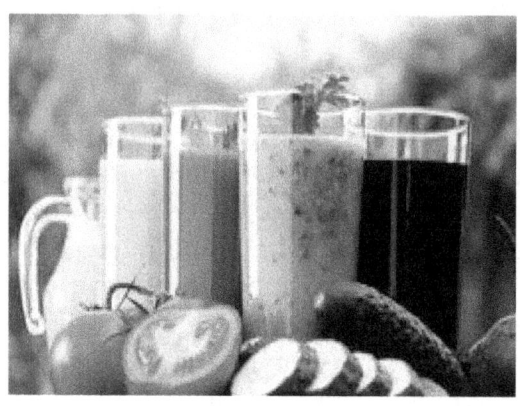

How To Apply Juicing To Your Detox Process

How that translates to detoxification

When juicing days or detoxification is used properly, the body is ridden of waste material that may build up over a period of time. Fluids pass through the body quite quickly and are excreted equally as quickly. Toxins, such as alcohol, however, can remain in the body as particles in the cells, such as cellulite and fat. The cell becomes stretched and the telltale signs of cellulite appear.

Detox does not have to be simply not eating or drinking only juices. Massage is also a detoxification procedure. Done properly it can break up these cells and release the toxins from the cell. Drinking fluids for a day can also release toxins from the cell as the body looks for other sources of food.

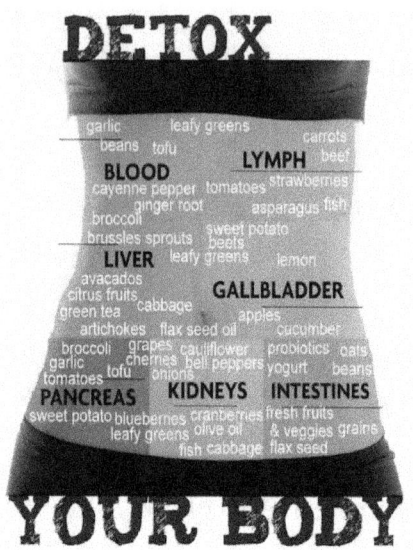

Detoxifying Ingredients And Home Remedies

There are a lot of home ingredients that can work double as cleansing and detoxifying juices if you simply put them through a juicer and drink the juice. Some of them are leafy green vegetables such as kale and cabbage, spinach, apples, most types of fruit, all of the berries varieties, cucumbers, and beets, to name a few.

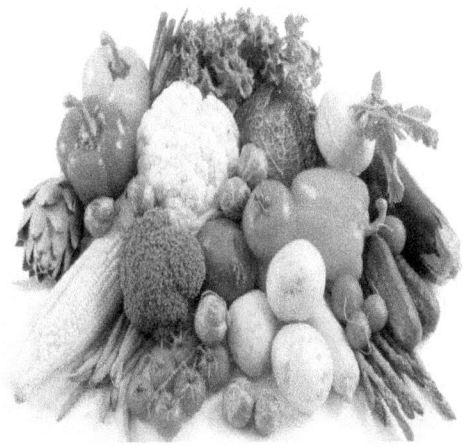

Some of these will end up as quite smooth juices, but the addition of small pieces of roughage in the way of pulp can only aid in the detoxifying effect. So when you are making your juices, don't worry if they are not completely smooth. Or you can turn these vegetables and fruit into smoothies, the better to access the nutrients held therein. With juicing, the only restriction is your imagination, so include ginger, herbs and spices to taste and whatever takes your fancy as long as it belongs in the fruit or vegetable varieties. Potatoes do not provide a very good juice, but this can be overcome by adding herbs or small sections of other vegetables such as broccoli.

If you want to juice, but your budget is tight, simply juice what is in season and add various seasonings to improve the flavor. You can also make delicious snacks with juicers from recipes that often come with the machine.

For instance, if kale, the new wonder vegetable is scarce and expensive, use spinach or cabbage or a leafy green that is in season and add pepper or some herb to it to make up the drink.

CHAPTER 8
Natural Body Detox –The old fashioned way vs. supplements (i.e., colon cleanse)

Not so long ago, it was the fashion in certain circles to undergo a colon cleanse regularly. The late Princess Diana swore to keep her figure and keep her metabolism in peak condition used detox. A colon cleanse can be either done naturally by the use of supplements or powders, or it can be achieved by having gallons of water inserted into the rectum and lower colon by a modified hose. The procedure is messy, but works, if the client can stand it for as long as it takes to return clear water, and is still used in certain clinics today.

This procedure removed a great deal of gunk. It also was unnatural and fell out of favor with many of those who underwent it for powders and pills that allowed the person to regulate to some degree what happened. Many people also thought that it was unnatural to keep stretching the colon with a hose and water, which may or may not have had ordinary soap added. Doctors also supposed that the sphincter to the lower bowel would lose its power.

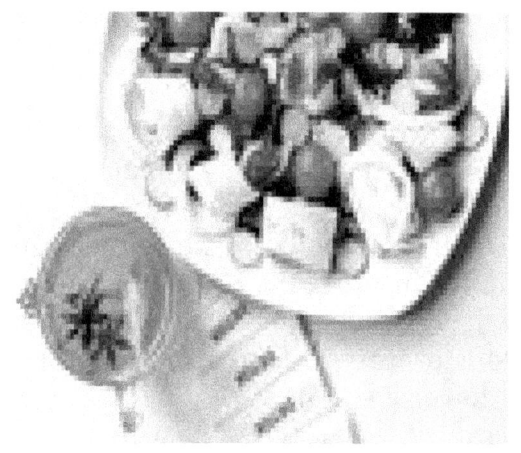

Either method removed or detoxified the colon or lower bowel, but are invasive and the person involved has very little control over them. Even today, pills and potions can often leave a person cut short on their way to a bathroom.

CHAPTER 9
FAQs/Final Thoughts

I thought I would finish off this eBook with some final thoughts on detoxification and juicing, and add a few questions and answers that are common in FAQs.

Again, I ask any of you who are planning a detoxification event or a juicing day to check with your health practitioner or doctor before you commence. This is only common sense.

Both of these procedures in my opinion are necessary if we wish to live healthy life. All through history, people who have lead healthy lives have made time to use detox in one way or another to cope with the demands of their existences. As has been pointed out, juicing has long been part of a healthy start to the day, whether it is continued for the rest of the day or not. A day of natural juices can kickstart the metabolism and reset it for returning to basic food consumption.

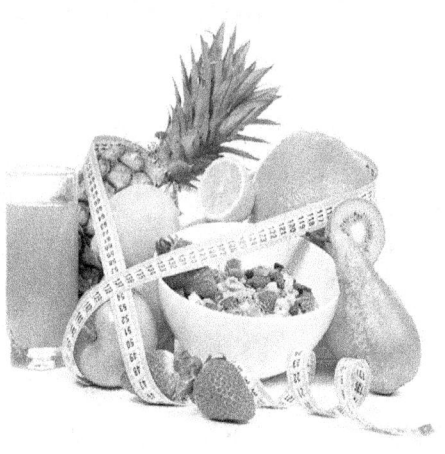

Detoxing is a part of many people's lives, which has been enforced on them to combat the excesses they have indulged in, to help them lead productive lives. In many times, it has enabled them to live quite long lives if continued. Detoxing can be simple, such as stopping smoking or it can be complicated and involve rearranging one's eating habits and patterns and including exercise. Any move that works to remove a toxin from the body is considered to be a part of detoxing.

FAQ

Who should have a detox?

Although the body can cleanse itself very well without any help usually occasionally things do overcome its systems. Constipation is one sign that the body is overwhelmed. People who suffer from this problem frequently may find a detoxing regime helpful. They may also find a juicing day beneficial if they cannot face a detox regime.

Is having a detox going to harm me?

No treatment is completely safe, which is why I strongly recommend you check with your doctor or health practitioner before commencing anything different to your usual routine. Juicing days or detox is not a usual activity, so it may result in some unexpected things occurring. Most detoxes and juicing days however do not do any more than help

with your health and leave you refreshed
and cleansed.

MORE FROM AUTHOR

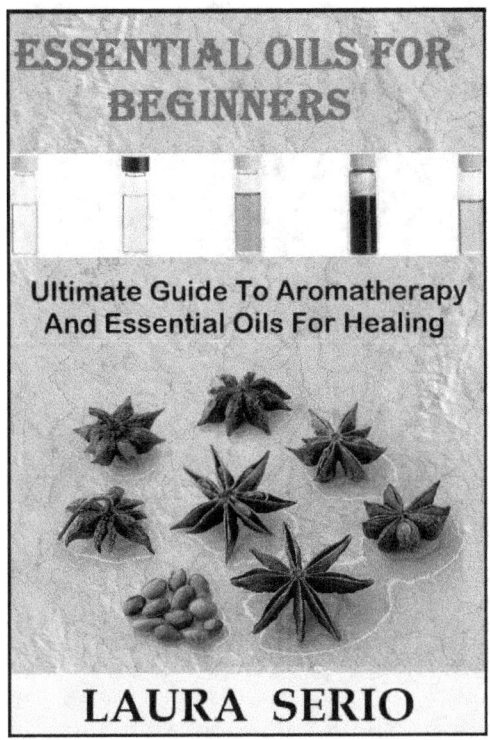

Essential Oils For Beginners

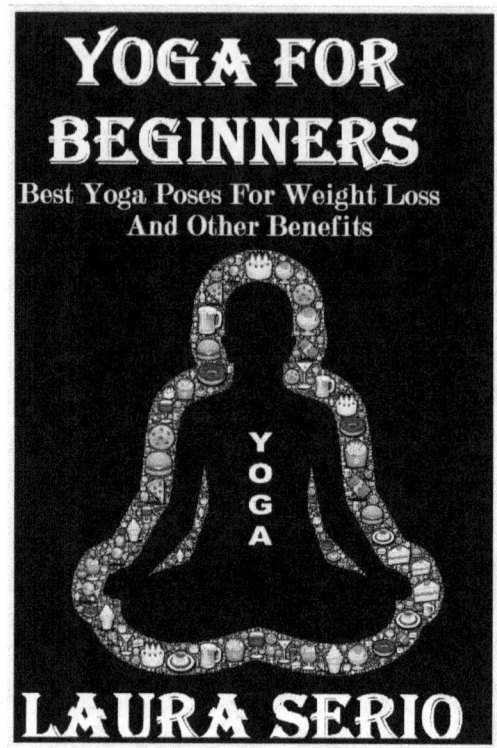

Yoga For Beginners

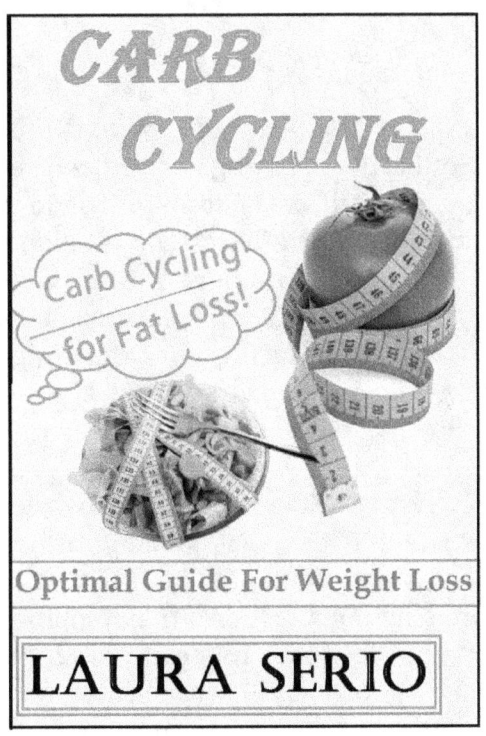

Carb Cycling

DISCLAIMER

This book cannot cover all the ins and outs of detoxing or indeed even juicing as well as it should. To do that would take maybe hundreds of chapters. All I am trying to do here is to give you a brief taste of what you can expect and why I think juicing or detoxing is worthwhile investigating from a point of health view.

I am NOT a medical professional, so I stress most seriously that you consult a health professional or your doctor before starting a fast or a major change to your diet. Not to do this can risk undoing all the good you are trying to do, especially if you are on prescribed medications. Some medications need proper food of some type to work or even to ensure they do not cause another problem. So do, please, consult your doctor BEFORE you start any change.

The information in this publication is complete and true to the best of our precise knowledge. Neither the publisher